Everything
Flax

Everything
Flax

EDITED BY LINDA BRAUN

more than 100 easy ways to work flax into your everyday diet

whitecap

Saskatchewan Flax Development Commission
A5A – 116 – 103rd Street East
Saskatoon, SK Canada S7N 1Y7
Telephone: (306) 664-1901
Email: saskflax@saskflax.com
Website: www.saskflax.com

The Saskatchewan Flax Development Commission, established
in 1996, represents over 12,000 flax producers in Saskatchewan.
A check-off system allows the Commission to direct and support
research, communication and market-facilitation programs
to promote and enhance flax production and value-added flax
products.

Whitecap Books is known for its expertise in the cookbook market,
and has produced some of the most innovative and familiar titles
found in kitchens across North America. Visit our website at
www.whitecap.ca.

Recipe development and testing: LeeAnn Bodnaryk, Linda Braun,
Gerald Henriksen, Mary Orr, Shona Pearson, N. Lee Pengilly
Food styling: LeeAnn Bodnaryk, Linda Braun, Leslie Sanders
Photography: Jerry Humeny, Black Box Images, Saskatoon, SK
Nutrient analysis: College of Pharmacy and Nutrition, University
of Saskatchewan, Saskatoon, SK
Project co-ordination: Linda Braun
Editing: Lesley Cameron
Design: Setareh Ashrafologhalai
Proofreading: Paula Ayer

Printed in Canada

Library and Archives Canada Cataloguing in Publication

Braun, Linda, 1955–

   Everything flax : more than 100 easy ways to work flax into
your everyday diet / Linda Braun.

Includes index.
ISBN 978-1-55285-981-0

   1. Cookery (Flaxseed). 2. Flaxseed in human nutrition. I. Title.

TX814.5.S44B73 2009   641.6'352   C2008-905578-0

The publisher acknowledges the financial support of the
Government of Canada through the Book Publishing Industry
Development Program (BPIDP) and the Province of British
Columbia through the Book Publishing Tax Credit.

09 10 11 12 13   5 4 3 2 1

Dear Reader

Saskatchewan flax producers work closely with Mother Nature and the vast prairie landscape to produce the world's best flax for today's health-conscious consumers.

Flaxseed in a balanced diet contributes essential fatty acids, particularly alpha-linolenic; generous amounts of soluble and insoluble fibre; lignans; protein; and essential vitamins and minerals.

The Saskatchewan Flax Development Commission is very pleased to present this collection of recipes, designed for all who recognize and value flaxseed as one component of a healthy lifestyle. The recipes are very tasty and have mass appeal. Our culinary team, who developed this collection, paid special attention to culinary trends, the availability of ingredients and the diverse tastes of people in communities across North America. Keep in mind that these recipes can be customized to your individual taste.

SaskFlax, representing over 12,000 Saskatchewan flax farmers, is proud to share these recipes and flax information, designed to help you make the most of what a healthy life has to offer.

Allen Kuhlmann, Chair
Saskatchewan Flax Development Commission

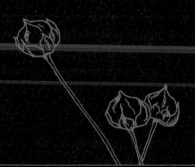

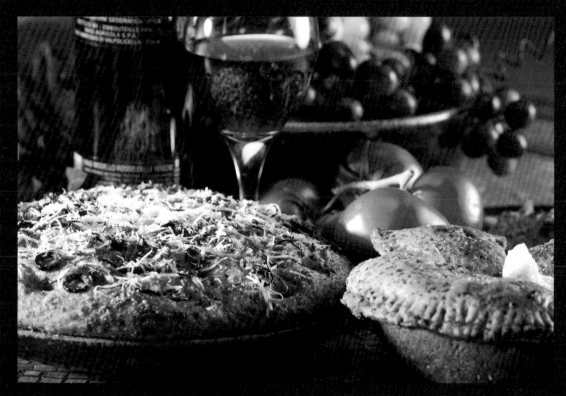

Pictured: *Onion & Olive Focaccia* (page 62) and *Veggie Calzones* (page 152)

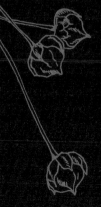

Contents

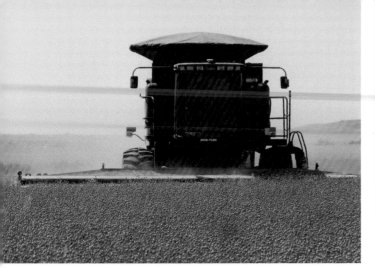
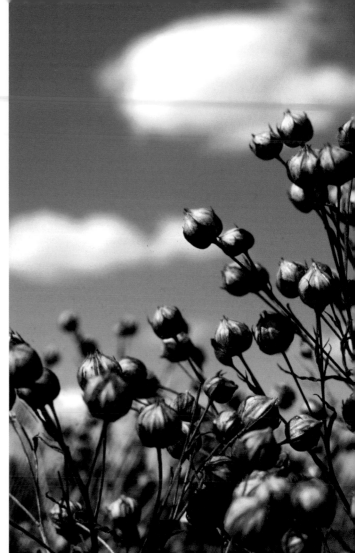
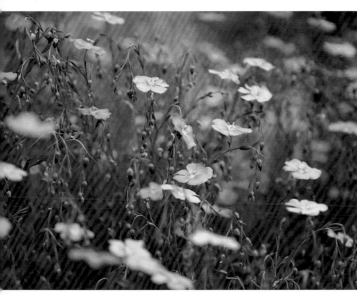
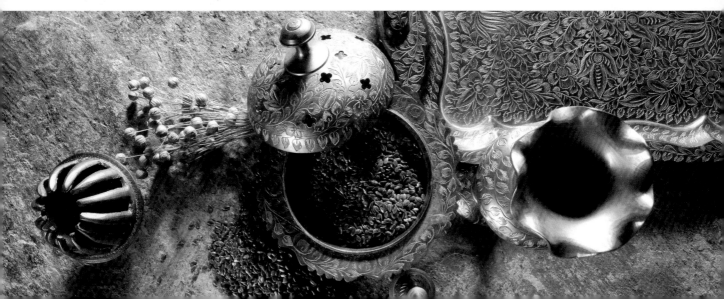

Introduction

BENEFITS OF FLAX IN THE DIET

Healthy eating and exercise are important for how we look and feel and how much we enjoy life. Making smart choices throughout our lives is thought to help reduce the risk of such conditions as heart disease, certain cancers, diabetes, osteoporosis and hypertension. While we all realize that taking measures to reduce our risk of some of these nutritional- and lifestyle-related conditions does not guarantee prevention, there is increasing scientific evidence that flax may help prevent heart disease, protect against inflammatory disorders and some cancers, and lower cholesterol.

Great nutrition starts with what you choose to ingest. You need carbohydrates, protein, fats, vitamins, minerals and water, but you also need to know the healthiest ways to find these basics. Fad diets come and go, but the general dietary advice of health professionals and experts remains relatively constant and basic: "Eat a wide variety of foods. Eat regularly and maintain a healthy body weight. Eat plenty of fruits and vegetables. Choose healthy carbohydrates. Drink plenty of fluids. Know and understand the difference between good fats and bad fats. Use salt in moderation!"

Flax has been prized for centuries for its nutritional and medicinal properties, and current scientific research appears to support many of the claims about its health benefits. Canada is fortunate to be home to many high-calibre researchers and the flax industry is proud to work with them. Research results are greeted with excitement and anticipation, as they increasingly not only validate some of the traditional uses of flaxseed, but also lead to the exploration of expanded uses aimed at improving our health and well-being. For more detailed information on scientific studies, visit the flax websites listed on page 5 and 232.

Flax is added to countless food products and functional foods because of the omega-3 fatty acids, lignans and fibre contained in the seed. And, as you will see from the recipes in this book, adding flax to your diet to gain health benefits has never been easier or tastier. Flax delivers!

FLAX AND NUTRITION

Flaxseed possesses a very healthy fatty acid profile:

Total Fat	42%
Polyunsaturates	30%
Omega-3	24%
Omega-6	6%
Monounsaturates	8%
Saturates	4%

Of the nutritionally beneficial polyunsaturates, approximately 16 percent is linolenic acid (LA), an omega-6 fatty acid, and approximately 57 percent is primarily alpha-linolenic acid (ALA), an omega-3 fatty acid.

Lignans are phytoestrogens that may affect our metabolism of hormones. The major lignan in flaxseed is secoisolariciresinol diglucoside (SDG), which exhibits antioxidant properties of potential benefit for some chronic diseases such as diabetes and high cholesterol.

Fibre, both soluble and insoluble, constitutes approximately 28 percent of the flaxseed. It exhibits positive effects on cholesterol, blood glucose and regularity.

Protein found in flaxseed is very similar to soybean protein. It is important for vegetarians relying on plant sources to meet their daily protein requirements.

RECOMMENDED DAILY INTAKE OF FLAXSEED AND FLAXSEED OIL

Flaxseed (whole or ground) 1 to 2 Tbsp (15 to 25 mL) of ground flaxseed (approximately 1 oz/25 g) may provide adequate supplementation of both ALA and lignans.

Flaxseed oil 2 to 3 grams of flaxseed oil, equivalent to 2 to 3 softgels (1,000 mg each) or about ½ tsp (2 mL) oil.

These recommendations are based on an average daily intake of 2,500 calories and Health Canada's recommended nutrient intake, which specifies that the minimum daily intake of ALA should be 0.5 percent of total energy.

It should be noted that nutrients from ground flaxseed are more readily available to the body. Careful chewing is strongly recommended to shred the whole flaxseed and release its nutrients.

ADDING FLAX TO YOUR DAILY DIET

- Add whole or ground flaxseed to baked goods such as breads, quick breads, muffins, cookies, pizza crust, meat loaf, casseroles or lasagna.
- Sprinkle whole or ground flaxseed on hot or cold cereal.
- Mix 2 Tbsp (25 mL) ground flaxseed into yogurt, ice cream, pudding or cottage cheese.
- Add flaxseed (whole or ground) to stews, spaghetti sauces, rice dishes, scrambled eggs, pancakes and waffles.

FLAX PRODUCTS IN THE MARKETPLACE

Ongoing research confirms that our society needs to be more mindful of health and that good health begins with the foods we eat. The food industry has recognized this need and products containing flax and flaxseed oil are gaining an ever-increasing market share. As well, omega-3-enhanced products such as eggs and meat are created by feeding diets rich in flax to birds and other animals.

Thanks to innovations in the food industry, we can now enjoy flax products such as:

- Non-hydrogenated margarines with flaxseed oil
- Omega-3-enriched yogurt and fruit juices
- Omega-3-enriched pork products and eggs
- Flax-based cold and hot cereals
- Flax-based breads, buns and bagels
- Flax-based muffins, pancakes and waffles
- Flax-based energy bars, granola and crackers

FLAX FACTS

Flaxseed Nutritional Analysis*

Note: A range of values is provided to reflect differences in the nutrient content of flaxseed due to environmental effects, such as temperature and rainfall, on seed development.

Nutrients	
Calories	492.0 kcal/100 g
	g/100 g
Total fat	34.0–42.0
Saturated fat	3.2–4.0
Polyunsaturated fat	22.4–30.0
Linoleic acid	4.3–6.0
Alpha-linolenic acid	18.1–24.0
Monounsaturated fat as oleic	6.9–8.0
Total carbohydrates	34.0–38.0
Fibre	28.0
Protein	21.0
Vitamins	
Tocopherols/vitamin E	5.0 mg ATE**/100 g
	mg/100 g
Ascorbic acid/vitamin C	0.50–1.30
Thiamin/vitamin B1	0.17–0.53
Riboflavin/vitamin B2	0.16–0.20
Niacin/nicotinic acid	1.40–3.21
Pyridoxine/vitamin B6	0.50–0.90
Pantothenic acid	0.57–1.50
	microg/kg
Folic acid	112.0–278.0
Biotin	6.0

Minerals	
	mg/100 g
Calcium	199.0–236.0
Copper	1.0
Iron	5.0–6.2
Magnesium	362.0–421.0
Manganese	3.0–3.2
Phosphorus	498.0–622.0
Potassium	681.0–831.0
Sodium	27.0–34.0
Zinc	4.2–5.0
	microg/100 g
Selenium	5.0
	mg/kg
Aluminum	3.00
Barium	2.00
Cadmium	0.25
Chromium	<1.00
Cobalt	0.17
Lead	<0.25
Molybdenum	<0.50
Nickel	1.70
Tin	<3.00

Weight and Calorie Content of Flaxseed (per specific measurement)

Ground Flaxseed					
1 cup (250 mL)	=	4.6 oz (130 g)	=	585 calories
1 Tbsp (15 mL)	=	0.3 oz (8 g)	=	36 calories
1 tsp (5 mL)	=	0.095 oz (2.7 g)	=	12 calories

Whole Flaxseed					
1 cup (250 mL)	=	6.3 oz (180 g)	=	810 calories
1 Tbsp (15 mL)	=	0.4 oz (11 g)	=	50 calories
1 tsp (5 mL)	=	0.14 oz (4 g)	=	18 calories

*Table adapted from USDA Nutrient Data Laboratory website (www.ars.usda.gov) with additional information from *Flaxseed: Health, Nutrition and Functionality* by Marion Vaisey-Genser and Diane H. Morris (Winnipeg, MB: Flax Council of Canada, 1994).

**Vitamin E values are given in ATEs (alpha-tocopherol equivalents): 1 mg alpha-tocopherol = 1 mg ATE × 0.8 mg alpha-tocopherol/mg ATE.

There are two types of flaxseed: brown and yellow (sometimes referred to as golden). Both contain the same nutritional benefits in terms of ALA, lignans, protein and dietary fibre.

Brown-seeded flax is the most widely grown in Canada. The yellow variety is currently grown under contract. Only certain farmers and companies have been granted licences to grow it. Which seed you consume is a matter of personal choice.

One other type of flaxseed, called "solin," resembles yellow flaxseed but is actually a derivative of flax. It has a much different nutrient profile, in particular much lower ALA levels, and is used primarily for frying. It is not available in seed form for consumers.

Flaxseed is available whole, ground, toasted whole, toasted ground and in oil form.

STORING FLAX

Whole flaxseed   High-quality, clean, dry whole flaxseed can be stored at room temperature for a year.

Ground flaxseed   Store ground flaxseed in an airtight, opaque container and refrigerate for up to 90 days. Freeze for up to a year. Frozen ground flaxseed does not need to be thawed before using.

Flaxseed oil   Store flaxseed oil in an airtight, opaque container and refrigerate. Most manufacturers recommend using flax oil within 6 to 8 weeks of opening.

BAKING WITH FLAXSEED

- Measure ground flaxseed loosely (do not pack) for baking. To grind flax at home, you can process small amounts in a food processor, blender or coffee grinder to achieve a free-flowing granular consistency (a texture similar to wheat bran). Grinding flax releases nutrients effectively, allowing you to absorb them more readily than from the whole seed.
- Try substituting ground flaxseed for fat in recipes at a ratio of three to one. For example, 1½ cups (375 mL) ground flaxseed can replace ½ cup (125 mL) butter, margarine or shortening. Baked goods will brown more quickly.
- Substitute 1 Tbsp (15 mL) ground flaxseed mixed with 3 Tbsp (45 mL) water for each egg required in a recipe.
- Substitute ground flaxseed for 25 percent of the flour in a recipe. However, note that this may result in a lower-volume baked good (that is, it may not rise as much as you would expect because flax doesn't have the same gluten content as wheat does) with a chewier texture.
- Substitute coarsely ground flaxseed for crushed nuts as a topping or coating ingredient for cookies.

COOKING WITH FLAXSEED OIL

- Flaxseed oil requires refrigeration to maintain its quality.
- Integrate flaxseed oil into your diet by using it in salad dressings, dips and spreads.
- Flaxseed oil is not recommended for frying, as it may undergo thermal oxidation when exposed to high temperatures and cause "off" flavours and odours.
- Make flaxseed butter/margarine by adding ½ cup (125 mL) flaxseed oil to ½ cup (125 mL) softened butter or margarine.

ROASTING/TOASTING FLAXSEED

- To roast flaxseed, place it in a single layer on a baking sheet in a 350°F (180°C) oven for 3 to 4 minutes. Cool in the baking sheet.
- To toast flaxseed, place whole flaxseed in a long-handled medium skillet. Cover securely. Hold over

high heat, shaking constantly until the flaxseed produces popping sounds. Remove from the heat and uncover when the popping ceases.

- Roasting/toasting flaxseed prevents the mucilage from being released, so roasted/toasted flaxseed won't act as a thickening agent in a recipe.
- Roasted/toasted flaxseed makes a great garnish for soups, stews and salads and a tasty topping for breakfast cereals, yogurt and fresh fruit.

INTERNET RESOURCES

There are several good North American websites about flax:

www.saskflax.com   www.fc2015.ca

www.flaxcouncil.ca   www.roastedflax.com

www.ameriflax.com   www.bioriginal.com

www.healthyflax.com

A WORD ABOUT THE RECIPES

- These recipes have been tested in both metric and imperial. Choose one system and stick to it throughout the recipe. Don't use a combination of both.
- Before starting, read the recipe completely. Then read it through again.
- Check for doneness at the earliest time specified in the recipe.
- These recipes are developed for general tastes; seasonings are an individual choice. Feel free to adjust seasonings to your taste!
- Some recipes call for different fat percentages in milk. Using your preferred choice (e.g., whole milk versus 1%) won't affect the recipe's success, but it will affect the nutritional content.
- Olive oil in recipes may be replaced with your favourite oil (i.e., canola, sunflower) with no effect on the recipe quality.
- Oats are available in a variety of forms which allows you to vary the texture and fibre content of many recipes. Rolled oats or old-fashioned oats are oat groats that have been steamed or flattened. They take about 15 minutes to cook. Quick-cooking oats are flattened thinner, making them faster to cook than rolled oats. Instant oats are made by cutting and precooking the oat groats prior to rolling. Steel-cut oats are groats that have been cut but not rolled.

- Unbleached and all-purpose flour may be used interchangeably.
- All recipes were tested using rimless baking sheets.
- Unless otherwise stated in the recipe, baked goods were baked in the bottom third of the oven.
- The nutrient analysis is based on using the first ingredient listed. Optional ingredients are not included in the calculations.
- The breakdown to saturated, monounsaturated and poly-unsaturated fats may not add up to the total fat due to other fatty acid components such as glycerol and trans fats.
- When recipes call for chicken or vegetable stocks or broths, you may use low-sodium versions if you prefer. This will reduce the sodium content of the dish.
- The term "pinch" as used in this book means the amount of a dry ingredient that you can pick up between your thumb and forefinger, approximately $\frac{1}{16}$ tsp (0.25 mL). The term "dash" means the amount of a liquid ingredient that can be dispensed from a bottle with a quick downward shake of your hand, approximately $\frac{1}{16}$ to $\frac{1}{8}$ tsp (0.25 to 0.5 mL).

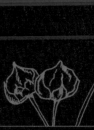

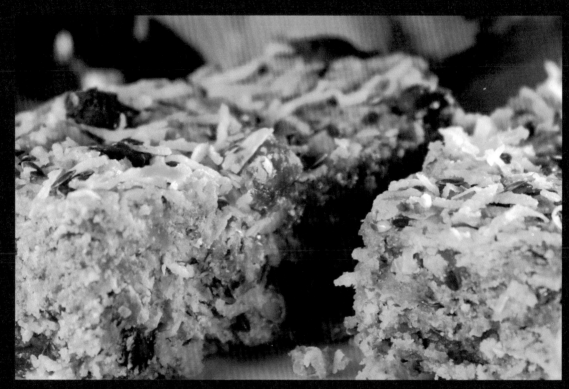

Pictured: *Flax Health Bars* (page 33)

Muffins, Loaves & Breakfast

Muffins, loaves, biscuits and scones are quick breads—they're relatively quick and easy to prepare. The use of baking powder, baking soda or a combination of the two rather than yeast allows for immediate rising when moisture and heat are added. Quick breads can be divided into two groups: batter breads, like the Cran-Orange Muffins, which are baked in molds (i.e., loaf and muffin tins); and quick dough breads, like the Granola Scones, which are stiff enough to hold their shape.

The recipes for these baked goods are not intimidating by any standard. Simply measure, add wet to dry, place in the pan, bake and enjoy!

Flaxseed, whether whole, ground or in oil form, is easy to incorporate and adds nutritional benefits such as protein, fibre and essential fatty acids to these familiar and appealing baked goods.

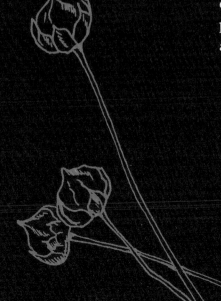

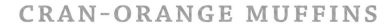

CRAN-ORANGE MUFFINS

2 cups (500 mL) fresh or frozen
 cranberries, chopped
⅓ cup (75 mL) granulated sugar
¾ cup (175 mL) orange juice
1 Tbsp (15 mL) orange zest
1 egg
2 cups (500 mL) unbleached
 all-purpose flour

¾ cup (175 mL) granulated sugar
½ cup (125 mL) ground flaxseed
1 tsp (5 mL) baking powder
½ tsp (2 mL) baking soda
½ tsp (2 mL) salt

YIELD: 12 muffins

NUTRIENT VALUES PER
SERVING (1 MUFFIN)

Calories	189
Protein	4.0 g
Carbohydrates	39.0 g
Fibre	2.9 g
Fat	2.9 g
Saturated	1.1 g
Monounsaturated	0.8 g
Polyunsaturated	0.8 g
Cholesterol	16.0 mg
Folate	40.0 mcg
Potassium	110 mg
Sodium	152 mg

1. Preheat the oven to 350°F (180°C). Spray a 12-cup muffin tin with non-stick cooking spray.
2. In a bowl, combine the cranberries, ⅓ cup (75 mL) sugar, orange juice, orange zest and egg.
3. In a separate bowl, combine the flour, ¾ cup (175 mL) sugar, ground flaxseed, baking powder, baking soda and salt.
4. Combine the cranberry mixture with the flour mixture until just blended.
5. Fill the muffin cups half to two-thirds full.
6. Bake for 10 to 20 minutes or until a wooden toothpick inserted in the centre of a muffin comes out clean.
7. Remove from the oven and cool in the tin for 5 minutes. Remove the muffins from the tin and transfer to a rack to cool completely.

These can be stored in an airtight container for up to 2 days or frozen for up to 2 months.

BRAN MUFFINS

2¼ cups (550 mL) unbleached
   all-purpose flour
1 cup (250 mL) granulated sugar
1 cup (250 mL) All-Bran cereal
¼ cup (50 mL) ground flaxseed
2 tsp (10 mL) baking powder

2 tsp (10 mL) baking soda
1 tsp (5 mL) salt
2 eggs
2 cups (500 mL) 1% milk
¾ cup (175 mL) canola oil
2 cups (500 mL) raisins

YIELD: 24 muffins

NUTRIENT VALUES PER
SERVING (1 MUFFIN)

Calories	204
Protein	3.5 g
Carbohydrates	31.5 g
Fibre	2.2 g
Fat	8.3 g
Saturated	1.0 g
Monounsaturated	4.4 g
Polyunsaturated	2.3 g
Cholesterol	16 mg
Folate	24 mcg
Potassium	196 mg
Sodium	266 mg

1. Preheat the oven to 350°F (180°C). Lightly spray two 12-cup muffin tins with non-stick cooking spray.
2. In a large bowl, combine the flour, sugar, All-Bran, ground flaxseed, baking powder, baking soda, salt, eggs, milk, oil and raisins. Mix well.
3. Fill the prepared muffin tins two-thirds full.
4. Bake for 18 to 20 minutes or until a wooden toothpick inserted in the centre of a muffin comes out clean.
5. Remove from the oven and cool in the tins for 5 minutes. Remove the muffins from the tins and transfer to a rack to cool completely.

These can be stored in an airtight container for up to 2 days or frozen for up to 2 months.

APPLE BRAN MUFFINS

Flax Fact: In the eighth century, Charlemagne of France made his feelings about the health benefits of eating flax perfectly clear when he passed a law that enforced its consumption.

1 cup (250 mL) buttermilk (see page 18)

½ cup (125 mL) lightly packed brown sugar

¼ cup (50 mL) canola oil

3 Tbsp (45 mL) fancy molasses

1 egg

1 cup (250 mL) natural wheat bran

1 cup (250 mL) unbleached all-purpose flour

½ cup (125 mL) ground flaxseed

1 tsp (5 mL) baking soda

½ tsp (2 mL) baking powder

½ tsp (2 mL) salt

1 cup (250 mL) finely chopped peeled and cored apple

¾ cup (175 mL) chopped pitted dates

YIELD: 12 muffins

NUTRIENT VALUES PER SERVING (1 MUFFIN)

Calories	211
Protein	4.3 g
Carbohydrates	35.8 g
Fibre	4.8 g
Fat	7.8 g
Saturated	1.6 g
Monounsaturated	3.6 g
Polyunsaturated	2.2 g
Cholesterol	16 mg
Folate	25 mcg
Potassium	332 mg
Sodium	249 mg

1. Preheat the oven to 400°F (200°C). Spray a 12-cup muffin tin with non-stick cooking spray.
2. In a large bowl, whisk together the buttermilk, brown sugar, canola oil, molasses and egg.
3. In another bowl, combine the bran, flour, flaxseed, baking soda, baking powder and salt.
4. Stir the dry ingredient mixture into the liquid ingredient mixture.
5. Stir in the chopped apple and dates.
6. Fill the muffin cups two-thirds full.
7. Bake for 17 minutes or until a wooden toothpick inserted in the centre of a muffin comes out clean.
8. Remove from the oven and cool in the tin for 5 minutes. Remove the muffins from the tin and transfer to a rack to cool completely.

These can be stored in an airtight container for up to 2 days or frozen for up to 2 months.

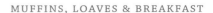

ORANGE BRAN FLAX MUFFINS

1½ cups (375 mL) oat bran

1 cup (250 mL) unbleached all-purpose flour

1 cup (250 mL) whole or ground flaxseed (see sidebar)

1 cup (250 mL) natural wheat bran

1 Tbsp (15 mL) baking powder

¼ tsp (1 mL) salt

2 whole oranges (washed, quartered, seeded)

1 cup (250 mL) lightly packed brown sugar

1 cup (250 mL) buttermilk (see page 18)

½ cup (125 mL) canola oil

2 eggs

1 tsp (5 mL) baking soda

1½ cups (375 mL) raisins (see sidebar)

YIELD: 18 muffins

NUTRIENT VALUES PER SERVING (1 MUFFIN)

Calories	275
Protein	6.1 g
Carbohydrates	44.5 g
Fibre	5.7 g
Fat	11.5 g
Saturated	1.4 g
Monounsaturated	4.0 g
Polyunsaturated	5.6 g
Cholesterol	24 mg
Folate	54 mcg
Potassium	439 mg
Sodium	236 mg

IF YOU ARE USING GROUND FLAXSEED, measure it first, then grind or mill it.

YOU CAN ALSO USE WHITE CHOCOLATE CHIPS instead of raisins.

1. Preheat the oven to 375°F (190°C). Place paper liners in the cups of three 6-cup muffin tins or spray 3 muffin tins with non-stick cooking spray.
2. In a large bowl, combine the oat bran, flour, flaxseed, wheat bran, baking powder and salt. Set aside.
3. In a blender or food processor, combine the orange quarters, brown sugar, buttermilk, oil, eggs and baking soda. Blend well.
4. Pour the orange mixture into the dry ingredients. Mix until well combined.
5. Stir in the raisins.
6. Fill the muffin cups almost to the top.
7. Bake for 18 to 20 minutes or until a wooden toothpick inserted in the centre of a muffin comes out clean.
8. Remove from the oven and cool in the tins for 5 minutes. Remove the muffins from the tins and transfer to a rack to cool completely.

These can be stored in an airtight container for up to 2 days or frozen for up to 2 months.

LOW-FAT BRAN MUFFINS

1½ cups (375 mL) natural wheat bran

1½ cups (375 mL) unbleached all-purpose flour

⅔ cup (150 mL) ground flaxseed

1 tsp (5 mL) baking soda

pinch salt

1 cup (250 mL) chopped dates

⅔ cup (150 mL) granulated sugar

¼ cup (50 mL) fancy molasses

2 Tbsp (25 mL) applesauce

2 eggs

1 cup (250 mL) soured skim milk (see page 17)

YIELD: 12 muffins

NUTRIENT VALUES PER SERVING (1 MUFFIN)

Calories	226
Protein	6.2 g
Carbohydrates	46.7 g
Fibre	6.8 g
Fat	4.4 g
Saturated	1.6 g
Monounsaturated	1.3 g
Polyunsaturated	1.2 g
Cholesterol	31 mg
Folate	36 mcg
Potassium	395 mg
Sodium	157 mg

1. Preheat the oven to 375°F (190°C). Spray a 12-cup muffin tin with non-stick cooking spray.
2. In a large bowl, combine the bran, flour, flaxseed, baking soda and salt. Stir in the dates to coat them.
3. In a separate bowl, whisk together the sugar, molasses, applesauce and eggs. Add the sour milk and stir to combine.
4. Add the liquid ingredients to the dry ingredients and mix lightly, until just moistened.
5. Fill the muffin cups two-thirds full.
6. Bake for 15 to 20 minutes or until a wooden toothpick inserted in the centre of a muffin comes out clean.
7. Remove from the oven and cool in the tin for 5 minutes. Remove the muffins from the tin and transfer to a rack to cool completely.

These can be stored in an airtight container for up to 2 days or frozen for up to 2 months.

CHEDDAR DILL MUFFINS

1½ cups (375 mL) unbleached
  all-purpose flour
½ cup (125 mL) ground golden
  flaxseed
2 Tbsp (25 mL) granulated sugar
1 Tbsp (15 mL) baking powder
½ tsp (2 mL) salt
¼ cup (50 mL) finely chopped
  fresh dill

1 cup (250 mL) low-fat plain yogurt
½ cup (125 mL) 1% milk
1 large egg, beaten
1 Tbsp (15 mL) flaxseed oil
½ cup (125 mL) grated aged
  cheddar cheese
1 Tbsp (15 mL) whole flaxseed

YIELD: 12 muffins

NUTRIENT VALUES PER
SERVING (1 MUFFIN)

Calories	140
Protein	6.2 g
Carbohydrates	18.7 g
Fibre	2.5 g
Fat	5.4 g
Saturated	2.5 g
Monounsaturated	1.5 g
Polyunsaturated	1.2 g
Cholesterol	22 mg
Folate	34 mcg
Potassium	145 mg
Sodium	220 mg

1. Preheat the oven to 400°F (200°C). Lightly spray a 12-cup muffin tin with non-stick cooking spray.
2. In a large bowl, combine the flour, ground flaxseed, sugar, baking powder and salt. Mix well.
3. Add the chopped dill and stir.
4. In another bowl, combine the yogurt, milk, beaten egg and flaxseed oil.
5. Add to the flour mixture and stir until just blended.
6. Fold in the grated cheese.
7. Fill the muffin cups three-quarters full.
8. Sprinkle the whole flaxseed overtop.
9. Bake for 18 to 20 minutes or until a wooden toothpick inserted into the centre of a muffin comes out clean.
10. Remove from the oven and cool in the tin for 5 minutes. Remove the muffins from the tin and transfer to a rack to cool completely.

These can be stored in an airtight container for up to 2 days or frozen for up to 2 months.

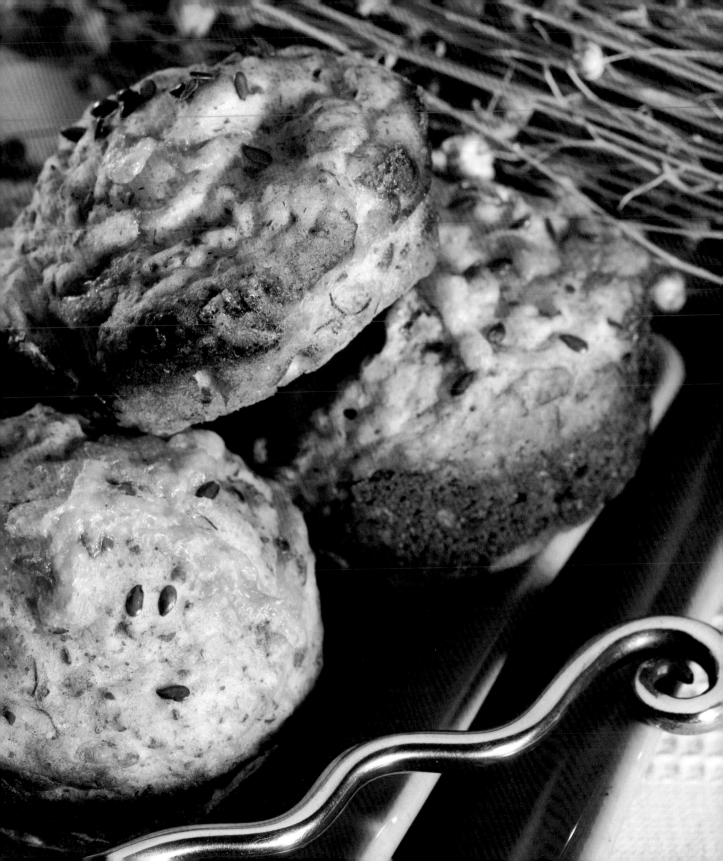

STRAWBERRY RHUBARB MUFFINS

Flax Fact: Vegetarians can substitute a flaxseed mixture for eggs in selected recipes like pancakes, muffins, and cookies. These baked goods are slightly gummier and chewier than normal, and the volume is decreased. When using the substitution formula, test a recipe first to determine if it meets your expectations.

Muffins

2 Tbsp (25 mL) canola oil

⅓ cup (75 mL) granulated sugar

2 large eggs

1 cup (250 mL) low-fat plain yogurt

2 cups (500 mL) unbleached all-purpose flour

⅔ cup (150 mL) ground flaxseed

1 tsp (5 mL) baking powder

1 tsp (5 mL) baking soda

½ tsp (2 mL) ground cinnamon

½ tsp (2 mL) salt

3 oz (90 g) package strawberry jelly powder

1 cup (250 mL) finely chopped rhubarb

Topping

2 Tbsp (25 mL) unbleached all-purpose flour

2 Tbsp (25 mL) granulated sugar

1 Tbsp (15 mL) butter or margarine

1 tsp (5 mL) whole flaxseed

YIELD: 12 muffins

NUTRIENT VALUES PER SERVING (1 MUFFIN)

Calories	104
Protein	3.1 g
Carbohydrates	16.7 g
Fibre	1.4 g
Fat	3.3 g
Saturated	1.2 g
Monounsaturated	1.3 g
Polyunsaturated	0.8 g
Cholesterol	11 mg
Folate	17 mcg
Potassium	70 mg
Sodium	138 mg

1. Preheat the oven to 350°F (180°C). Spray a 12-cup muffin tin with non-stick cooking spray.
2. For the muffins, in a bowl, whisk together the oil, sugar, eggs and yogurt until well blended.
3. In a separate bowl, mix together the flour, ground flaxseed, baking powder, baking soda, cinnamon and salt.
4. In a small bowl, combine the jelly powder and rhubarb.
5. Pour the liquid ingredients over the dry ingredients. Add the rhubarb mixture and stir until the dry ingredients are moistened.
6. Measure ⅓ cup (75 mL) of batter into each muffin cup.
7. For the topping, combine the flour, sugar, butter and whole flaxseed until the mixture resembles coarse crumbs. Sprinkle 1 tsp (5 mL) over each muffin.
8. Bake for 20 to 25 minutes or until a wooden toothpick inserted in the centre of a muffin comes out clean.
9. Remove from the oven and cool in the tin for 5 minutes. Remove the muffins from the tin and transfer to a rack to cool completely.

These can be stored in an airtight container for up to 2 days or frozen for up to 2 months.

CHOCOLATE ZUCCHINI MUFFINS

2½ cups (625 mL) unbleached
   all-purpose flour
¼ cup (50 mL) unsweetened cocoa
   powder
¼ cup (50 mL) ground flaxseed
1 tsp (5 mL) salt
1 tsp (5 mL) baking soda
½ tsp (2 mL) baking powder

1½ cups (375 mL) granulated sugar
½ cup (125 mL) margarine
¼ cup (50 mL) canola oil
2 eggs
½ cup (125 mL) soured 1% milk
   (see sidebar)
2 cups (500 mL) finely grated
   unpeeled zucchini

YIELD: 24 muffins

NUTRIENT VALUES PER
SERVING (1 MUFFIN)

Calories	174
Protein	2.7 g
Carbohydrates	25.3 g
Fibre	0.8 g
Fat	7.2 g
Saturated	1.2 g
Monounsaturated	2.7 g
Polyunsaturated	2.9 g
Cholesterol	18 mg
Folate	14 mcg
Potassium	85 mg
Sodium	223 mg

TO MAKE ½ CUP (125 ML)
OF SOUR MILK, measure
2 tsp (10 mL) vinegar into a
liquid measuring cup. Add
milk to the ½-cup (125 mL)
mark. Let stand for 5 minutes before using.

1. Preheat the oven to 350°F (180°C). Place paper liners into the cups of two 12-cup muffin tins.
2. In a bowl, combine the flour, cocoa powder, flaxseed, salt, baking soda and baking powder.
3. In a separate bowl, cream the sugar, margarine and oil.
4. Add the eggs and sour milk, mixing well.
5. Add the flour mixture, stirring until just mixed.
6. Add the zucchini and mix again.
7. Fill each paper cup half to two-thirds full.
8. Bake for 18 to 20 minutes or until a wooden toothpick inserted in the centre of a muffin comes out clean.
9. Remove from the oven and cool in the tins for 5 minutes. Remove the muffins from the tins and transfer to a rack to cool completely.

These can be stored in an airtight container for up to 2 days or frozen for up to 2 months.

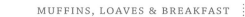

GOLDEN GRAIN MUFFINS

1 cup (250 mL) quick-cooking oats

½ cup (125 mL) natural wheat bran

½ tsp (2 mL) ground cinnamon

½ tsp (2 mL) salt

1 cup (250 mL) buttermilk
  (see sidebar)

1 whole egg

1 egg white

½ cup (125 mL) liquid honey

¼ cup (50 mL) canola oil

1 cup (250 mL) whole wheat flour

¾ cup (175 mL) ground flaxseed

2 tsp (10 mL) baking powder

1 tsp (5 mL) baking soda

½ cup (125 mL) golden raisins, chopped

1 tsp (5 mL) whole flaxseed (optional)

YIELD: 12 muffins

NUTRIENT VALUES PER
SERVING (1 MUFFIN)

Calories	225
Protein	6.4 g
Carbohydrates	35.1 g
Fibre	5.7 g
Fat	9.3 g
Saturated	2.2 g
Monounsaturated	4.0 g
Polyunsaturated	2.8 g
Cholesterol	16 mg
Folate	8 mcg
Potassium	256 mg
Sodium	284 mg

FOR A BUTTERMILK SUB-
STITUTE you can use 1 cup
(250 mL) plain yogurt, or mix
1 Tbsp (15 mL) lemon juice or
vinegar with enough milk to
equal 1 cup (250 mL). Let stand
for 5 minutes before using.

1. Preheat the oven to 375°F (190°C). Spray a 12-cup muffin tin with non-stick cooking spray.
2. In a large bowl, combine the oats, bran, cinnamon, salt and buttermilk. Mix well and let stand 15 minutes.
3. Beat the whole egg and egg white together. Add the egg mixture, honey and oil to the oat mixture. Mix well.
4. In another bowl, combine the whole wheat flour, flaxseed, baking powder and baking soda. Add to the oat mixture and stir just until moistened.
5. Stir in the raisins.
6. Measure ⅓ cup (75 mL) of batter into each muffin cup. Sprinkle with whole flaxseed if desired.
7. Bake for 18 to 20 minutes or until a wooden toothpick inserted in the centre of a muffin comes out clean.
8. Remove from the oven and cool in the tin for 5 minutes. Remove the muffins from the tin and transfer to a rack to cool completely.

These can be stored in an airtight container for up to 2 days or frozen for up to 2 months.

BANANA BREAD

Bread

1¾ cups (425 mL) unbleached all-purpose flour

1 cup (250 mL) ground flaxseed

¾ cup (175 mL) granulated sugar

1 tsp (5 mL) baking powder

½ tsp (2 mL) baking soda

½ tsp (2 mL) salt

1 cup (250 mL) mashed bananas

2 Tbsp (25 mL) canola oil

2 eggs

Topping

2 Tbsp (25 mL) chopped pecans

2 Tbsp (25 mL) brown sugar

½ tsp (2 mL) ground cinnamon

YIELD: 1 loaf (20 slices)

NUTRIENT VALUES PER SERVING (1 SLICE)

Calories	132
Protein	3.2 g
Carbohydrates	21.3 g
Fibre	2.4 g
Fat	5.0 g
Saturated	1.4 g
Monounsaturated	1.9 g
Polyunsaturated	1.4 g
Cholesterol	19 mg
Folate	22 mcg
Potassium	115 mg
Sodium	113 mg

1. Preheat the oven to 350°F (180°C). Spray an 8½- × 4½-inch (1.5 L) loaf pan with non-stick cooking spray.
2. For the bread, in a bowl, mix together the flour, flaxseed, sugar, baking powder, baking soda and salt.
3. In a separate bowl, beat together the bananas, oil and eggs.
4. Add the liquid ingredients to the dry ingredients. Stir only until the ingredients are moistened.
5. Pour into the prepared loaf pan.
6. For the topping, in a bowl, combine the pecans, brown sugar and cinnamon. Sprinkle over the batter in the loaf pan. Pat the topping down gently into the batter.
7. Bake for 55 minutes to 1 hour or until a wooden toothpick inserted in the centre of the bread comes out clean.
8. Remove from the oven and cool in the pan for 5 minutes before transferring to a rack to cool completely.

This can be stored in an airtight container for up to 2 days or frozen for up to 2 months.

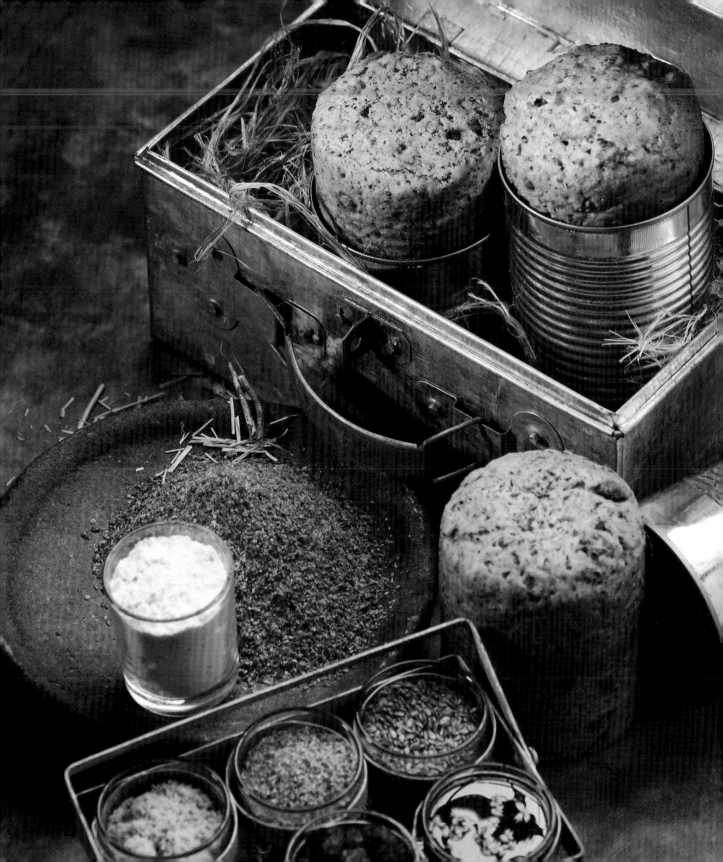

STEAMED BOSTON BREAD

1⅓ cups (325 mL) unbleached
all-purpose flour

1⅓ cups (325 mL) whole wheat flour

⅓ cup (75 mL) ground flaxseed

2 Tbsp (25 mL) brown sugar

1½ tsp (7 mL) salt

1 tsp (5 mL) baking powder

1 tsp (5 mL) baking soda

½ cup (125 mL) raisins, chopped

1⅔ cups (400 mL) water

¼ cup (50 mL) fancy molasses

YIELD: 3 loaves (each cut into 3 slices)

NUTRIENT VALUES PER SERVING (2 SLICES)

Calories	213
Protein	5.6 g
Carbohydrates	45.2 g
Fibre	4.5 g
Fat	2.6 g
Saturated	0.9 g
Monounsaturated	0.6 g
Polyunsaturated	0.8 g
Cholesterol	0 mg
Folate	41 mcg
Potassium	341 mg
Sodium	570 mg

1. Grease three 19 oz (540 mL) empty tin cans.
2. In a large bowl, combine both flours, the flaxseed, brown sugar, salt, baking powder and baking soda.
3. Add the raisins and toss to coat.
4. In a measuring cup, stir together the water and molasses.
5. Add to the dry ingredients. Stir until just combined.
6. Fill the tins two-thirds full.
7. Cover them with wax paper, then a layer of aluminum foil and secure with kitchen string.
8. Place the tins on a rack inside a large saucepan or Dutch oven.
9. Fill the saucepan or Dutch oven with boiling water to halfway up the tins. Cover with a lid.
10. Bring to a gentle simmer and steam for 2 hours.
11. Remove the bread from the tins.
12. Serve warm.

These can be stored in an airtight container for up to 2 days or frozen for up to 2 months.

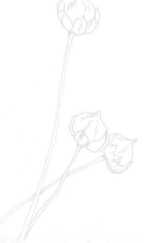

PEACH COFFEE CAKE

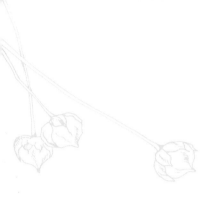

Base

¾ cup (175 mL) natural wheat bran

1 cup (250 mL) 1% milk

¼ cup (50 mL) granulated sugar

1 large egg

2 Tbsp (25 mL) flaxseed oil

1 cup (250 mL) unbleached
    all-purpose flour

¼ cup (50 mL) ground flaxseed

1 Tbsp (15 mL) baking powder

¼ tsp (1 mL) salt

Topping

14 oz (398 mL) can sliced peaches,
    drained

2 Tbsp (25 mL) brown sugar

2 Tbsp (25 mL) granulated sugar

1 Tbsp (15 mL) unbleached
    all-purpose flour

1½ tsp (7 mL) ground cinnamon

1 Tbsp (15 mL) flaxseed oil

YIELD: one 8-inch (20 cm)
square pan (9 pieces)

NUTRIENT VALUES PER
SERVING (1 PIECE)

Calories	180
Protein	4.8 g
Carbohydrates	30.2 g
Fibre	4.0 g
Fat	6.4 g
Saturated	1.3 g
Monounsaturated	1.4 g
Polyunsaturated	3.4 g
Cholesterol	25 mg
Folate	27 mcg
Potassium	187 mg
Sodium	244 mg

1. Preheat the oven to 375°F (190°C). Grease and flour an 8-inch (20 cm) square pan.
2. In a small bowl, soak the bran in the milk for 10 minutes.
3. In a large bowl, whisk together the sugar, egg and flaxseed oil.
4. In another bowl, stir together the flour, ground flaxseed, baking powder and salt.
5. Add the flour mixture, alternating with the bran mixture, to the sugar and egg mixture. Stir until the ingredients are just moistened.
6. Spread the batter into the prepared pan.
7. Lay the peaches in rows on top of the batter.
8. In a small bowl, mix together the brown and granulated sugars, flour and cinnamon.
9. Stir in the flaxseed oil until moistened.
10. Sprinkle the topping over the peaches.
11. Bake for 45 minutes or until a wooden toothpick inserted in the centre of the cake comes out clean.
12. Remove from the oven and cool on a rack.

Serve with a dollop of vanilla yogurt or whipped cream if desired. This can be stored in an airtight container for up to 2 days or frozen for up to 2 months.

FLAX SCONES

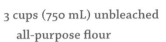

3 cups (750 mL) unbleached
   all-purpose flour
½ cup + 2 Tbsp (125 mL + 25 mL)
   whole flaxseed, divided
¼ cup (50 mL) lightly packed
   brown sugar
2 tsp + 1 Tbsp (10 mL + 15 mL)
   grated orange zest, divided

1 Tbsp (15 mL) baking powder
¾ tsp (4 mL) salt
¾ cup (175 mL) shortening
1 cup (250 mL) orange juice, divided
2 Tbsp (25 mL) granulated sugar

YIELD: 12 scones

NUTRIENT VALUES PER
SERVING (1 SCONE)

Calories	287
Protein	5.3 g
Carbohydrates	32.3 g
Fibre	3.5 g
Fat	16.6 g
Saturated	5.3 g
Monounsaturated	4.8 g
Polyunsaturated	5.9 g
Cholesterol	0 mg
Folate	49 mcg
Potassium	122 mg
Sodium	248 mg

1. Preheat the oven to 425°F (220°C). Spray a baking sheet with non-stick
   cooking spray.
2. In a large bowl, combine the flour, ½ cup (125 mL) of the flaxseed, the brown
   sugar, 2 tsp (10 mL) of the orange zest, the baking powder and salt.
3. Using a pastry blender or 2 knives, cut the shortening into the flour mixture
   until it resembles coarse crumbs.
4. Reserve 2 Tbsp (25 mL) of the orange juice. Add the remaining orange juice to the
   crumb mixture and mix lightly with a fork until the mixture forms a soft dough.
5. Put the dough on a lightly floured clean work surface and knead gently 4 to
   5 times.
6. Divide the dough in half and form each half into a ball. Roll each ball into a
   6-inch (15 cm) circle 1 inch (2.5 cm) thick.
7. Cut each ball into 6 wedges. Place the wedges on the prepared baking sheet.
8. Prick the tops of the wedges with a fork.
9. In a saucepan, heat the reserved orange juice and the granulated sugar to make
   a glaze. Bring to a boil, then remove from the heat. Add the remaining 1 Tbsp
   (15 mL) orange zest.
10. Brush the tops of the scones with the glaze, then sprinkle with the remaining
   2 Tbsp (25 mL) flaxseed. Reserve the remaining glaze.
11. Bake for 16 to 20 minutes or until brown. Remove from the oven and glaze the
   tops again with the reserved glaze.

*These can be stored in an airtight container for up to 2 days or frozen for up to
2 months.*

GRANOLA SCONES

Flax Fact: Mahatma Gandhi is credited with the observation that "Wherever flax seed becomes a regular food item among the people, there will be better health."

Scones

½ cup (125 mL) old-fashioned rolled oats

1 egg, beaten

⅔ cup (150 mL) buttermilk (see page 18)

1 tsp (5 mL) vanilla extract

¾ cup (175 mL) unbleached all-purpose flour

½ cup (125 mL) whole wheat flour

½ cup (125 mL) ground flaxseed

2 Tbsp (25 mL) granulated sugar

2 tsp (10 mL) baking powder

½ tsp (2 mL) baking soda

½ tsp (2 mL) ground cinnamon

½ tsp (2 mL) salt

⅓ cup (75 mL) butter or margarine

½ cup (125 mL) currants

¼ cup (50 mL) sliced almonds

2 Tbsp (25 mL) sunflower seeds

1 egg white

Topping

1 Tbsp (15 mL) sliced almonds

1 Tbsp (15 mL) quick-cooking oats

1 Tbsp (15 mL) raw sunflower seeds

1 tsp (5 mL) whole flaxseed

YIELD: 8 scones

NUTRIENT VALUES PER SERVING (1 SCONE)

Calories	311
Protein	9.2 g
Carbohydrates	35.1 g
Fibre	6.1 g
Fat	17.0 g
Saturated	3.3 g
Monounsaturated	6.7 g
Polyunsaturated	6.3 g
Cholesterol	24 mg
Folate	37 mcg
Potassium	323 mg
Sodium	433 mg

1. Preheat the oven to 375°F (190°C).
2. In a large bowl, combine the rolled oats, egg, buttermilk and vanilla. Let stand for 5 minutes.
3. In another large bowl, combine both flours, the ground flaxseed, sugar, baking powder, baking soda, cinnamon and salt.
4. Cut in the butter. Rub it in lightly with your fingertips until the mixture resembles coarse crumbs.
5. Stir in the currants, almonds and sunflower seeds.
6. Stir the buttermilk mixture into the dry ingredients and mix just until moistened.
7. Turn the dough onto a clean, floured work surface and knead 6 to 8 times. The dough will be sticky.
8. Flatten into an ungreased 8-inch (20 cm) round pan.
9. Whisk together the egg white and 1 Tbsp (15 mL) water. Brush over the dough.

10. Sprinkle with the almonds, quick-cooking oats, sunflower seeds and whole flaxseed. Score the dough into 8 wedges.
11. Bake for 25 to 30 minutes or until a wooden toothpick inserted in the centre comes out clean.
12. Remove from the oven and cool in the pan for 5 minutes. Remove the scones from the pan and separate along the score lines into 8 wedges. Serve warm.

These can be stored in an airtight container for up to 2 days or frozen for up to 3 months.

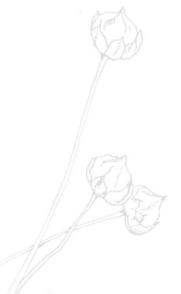

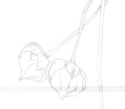

PUMPKIN CRANBERRY SCONES

Scones

1 cup (250 mL) unbleached
 all-purpose flour

½ cup (125 mL) whole wheat flour

⅓ cup (75 mL) ground flaxseed

¼ cup (50 mL) granulated sugar

1 Tbsp (15 mL) baking powder

1½ tsp (7 mL) pumpkin pie spice

¼ cup (50 mL) margarine, cold

½ cup (125 mL) canned pumpkin

⅓ cup (75 mL) cran-raisins

¼ cup (50 mL) raw, shelled
 pumpkin seeds

½ cup (125 mL) 1% milk

1 egg, beaten

Topping

1 tsp (5 mL) raw, shelled
 pumpkin seeds

1 tsp (5 mL) whole flaxseed

YIELD: 8 scones

NUTRIENT VALUES PER
SERVING (1 SCONE)

Calories	248
Protein	6.6 g
Carbohydrates	32.5 g
Fibre	4.2 g
Fat	11.5 g
Saturated	2.6 g
Monounsaturated	4.1 g
Polyunsaturated	4.2 g
Cholesterol	24 mg
Folate	37 mcg
Potassium	202 mg
Sodium	230 mg

1. Preheat the oven to 400°F (200°C). Line a baking sheet with parchment paper.
2. In a large bowl, combine both flours, the ground flaxseed, sugar, baking powder and pumpkin pie spice.
3. Cut in the margarine to form pea-sized pieces. Continue working the mixture by gently rubbing it with your fingers to create a mealy texture.
4. Add the pumpkin and rub it into the flour mixture with your fingers until the mixture resembles coarse crumbs. Stir in the cran-raisins and pumpkin seeds.
5. In a small bowl, combine the milk with the beaten egg. Reserve 2 Tbsp (25 mL) for the topping.
6. Add the remaining egg mixture to the flour mixture. Stir until the dough forms a very soft, sticky ball.
7. Place the dough on the prepared baking sheet. Flatten and shape the ball into an 8-inch (20 cm) disk. Score it into 8 wedges. Brush with the reserved egg mixture.
8. Lightly sprinkle the dough with the pumpkin seeds and whole flaxseed.
9. Bake for 25 to 30 minutes or until the scone is golden brown and a wooden toothpick inserted in the centre comes out clean.
10. Remove from the oven. Let the scone cool on a rack in the pan for 2 minutes, then separate it along the score lines into 8 wedges.

These can be stored in an airtight container for up to 2 days or frozen for up to 2 months. Pictured on page 114.

SAVOURY FLAX BISCUITS

2 cups (500 mL) unbleached
   all-purpose flour
2 Tbsp (25 mL) brown sugar
4 tsp (20 mL) baking powder
½ tsp (2 mL) salt
½ cup (125 mL) shortening
1 cup (250 mL) grated carrot

¼ cup (50 mL) coarsely ground flaxseed
2 tsp (10 mL) Mrs. Dash original
   seasoning or any salt-free herb
   and spice seasoning
⅔ cup (150 mL) 2% milk
1 egg, beaten

YIELD: 18 biscuits

NUTRIENT VALUES PER
SERVING (1 BISCUIT)

Calories	132
Protein	2.6 g
Carbohydrates	14.7 g
Fibre	1.0 g
Fat	7.0 g
Saturated	1.7 g
Monounsaturated	2.2 g
Polyunsaturated	2.0 g
Cholesterol	12 mg
Folate	N/A
Potassium	188 mg
Sodium	147 mg

1. Preheat the oven to 450°F (230°C).
2. In a large mixing bowl, sift together the flour, sugar, baking powder and salt.
3. Cut in the shortening until the mixture resembles coarse crumbs.
4. Stir in the carrot, flaxseed and seasoning.
5. Combine the milk and egg. Add this to the flour mixture all at once and stir until the dough forms a ball.
6. Turn the dough out onto a lightly floured clean work surface. Knead gently 20 times.
7. Roll the dough to a ¾-inch (2 cm) thickness and cut out biscuits with a 2-inch (5 cm) floured cookie cutter.
8. Place the biscuits 1 inch (2.5 cm) apart on an ungreased baking sheet.
9. Bake for 10 to 14 minutes or until golden brown.
10. Remove from the oven and transfer the biscuits to a rack to cool.

These can be stored in an airtight container for up to 2 days or frozen for up to 2 months.

SASKATOON BAKED BANNOCK

½ cup (125 mL) whole wheat flour

½ cup (125 mL) unbleached
   all-purpose flour

½ cup (125 mL) quick-cooking oats

¼ cup (50 mL) ground flaxseed

¼ cup (50 mL) whole flaxseed

2 Tbsp (25 mL) granulated sugar

2 tsp (10 mL) baking powder

½ tsp (2 mL) salt

½ cup (125 mL) fresh or thawed
   frozen Saskatoon berries

¾ cup (175 mL) water

2 Tbsp (25 mL) melted butter or
   margarine

YIELD: 6 wedges

NUTRIENT VALUES PER
SERVING (1 WEDGE)

Calories	217
Protein	6.4 g
Carbohydrates	31.0 g
Fibre	6.1 g
Fat	10.0 g
Saturated	2.9 g
Monounsaturated	3.3 g
Polyunsaturated	3.4 g
Cholesterol	0 mg
Folate	24 mcg
Potassium	190 mg
Sodium	341 mg

1. Preheat the oven to 400°F (200°C). Spray an 8-inch (20 cm) pie plate with non-stick cooking spray.
2. In a large bowl, combine both flours, the oats, ground and whole flaxseed, sugar, baking powder and salt.
3. Add the Saskatoon berries.
4. Drizzle the water and melted butter over the flour mixture, stir with a fork and add more water if needed to make a sticky dough.
5. Pat the dough into the prepared pie plate.
6. Bake for 20 to 25 minutes or until the bannock is golden brown and a wooden toothpick inserted in the centre comes out clean.
7. Remove from the oven and cut into 6 wedges.
8. Serve warm with butter, jam or Maple-Pecan Topping (page 123).

These can be stored in an airtight container for up to 2 days or frozen for up to 2 months.

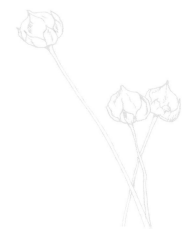

CORNBREAD LOAF

1½ cups (375 mL) buttermilk
   (see page 18)
¼ cup (50 mL) margarine, melted
2 Tbsp (25 mL) liquid honey
2 eggs
1½ cups (375 mL) cornmeal
¾ cup (175 mL) unbleached
   all-purpose flour

½ cup (125 mL) ground flaxseed
2 tsp (10 mL) baking powder
½ tsp (2 mL) baking soda
½ tsp (2 mL) salt
12 oz (355 mL) can whole kernel
   corn, drained

YIELD: 1 loaf (16 slices)

NUTRIENT VALUES PER
SERVING (1 SLICE)

Calories	149
Protein	4.3 g
Carbohydrates	21.3 g
Fibre	3.1 g
Fat	6.0 g
Saturated	1.5 g
Monounsaturated	2.1 g
Polyunsaturated	1.9 g
Cholesterol	24 mg
Folate	36 mcg
Potassium	116 mg
Sodium	286 mg

1. Preheat the oven to 375°F (190°C). Spray a 9- × 5-inch (2 L) loaf pan with non-stick cooking spray.
2. In a medium bowl, combine the buttermilk, melted margarine, honey and eggs. Blend well.
3. In another large bowl, combine the cornmeal, flour, ground flaxseed, baking powder, baking soda and salt.
4. Use a fork to stir the buttermilk mixture and corn into the cornmeal mixture just until moistened.
5. Spoon the batter into the prepared loaf pan.
6. Bake for 45 to 55 minutes or until a wooden toothpick inserted in the centre comes out clean.
7. Remove from the oven and cool in the loaf pan.

This can be stored in an airtight container for up to 2 days or frozen for up to 2 months.

PIZZA BREAD

½ cup (125 mL) sun-dried tomatoes

2¼ cups (550 mL) unbleached
   all-purpose flour

½ cup (125 mL) light Parmesan cheese

1 Tbsp (15 mL) granulated sugar

½ cup (125 mL) ground flaxseed

1 Tbsp (15 mL) baking powder

2 tsp (10 mL) crushed dried oregano

½ tsp (2 mL) salt

¼ tsp (1 mL) black pepper

1¼ cups (300 mL) skim milk

2 Tbsp (25 mL) canola oil

1 egg

1 small tomato, diced

¼ cup (50 mL) diced green bell pepper

⅓ cup (75 mL) shredded mozzarella
   cheese

YIELD: 1 loaf (20 slices)

NUTRIENT VALUES PER
SERVING (1 SLICE)

Calories	119
Protein	4.9 g
Carbohydrates	16.8 g
Fibre	1.6 g
Fat	3.9 g
Saturated	0.7 g
Monounsaturated	1.1 g
Polyunsaturated	1.9 g
Cholesterol	14 mg
Folate	24 mcg
Potassium	191 mg
Sodium	177 mg

TO MAKE PIZZA BREAD
MUFFINS, increase the milk
to 1½ cups (375 mL) and
reduce the flour to 2 cups
(500 mL). Bake for 25 minutes. (Yield: 12 muffins)

1. Cover the sun-dried tomatoes with boiling water. Let stand for 10 minutes or until softened. Drain and dice the tomatoes.
2. Preheat the oven to 350°F (180°C). Spray an 8½- × 4½-inch (1.5 L) loaf pan with non-stick cooking spray.
3. In a bowl, combine the rehydrated sun-dried tomatoes, flour, Parmesan cheese, sugar, flaxseed, baking powder, oregano, salt and pepper.
4. In a separate bowl, whisk together the milk, oil and egg.
5. Pour the liquid ingredients into the dry ingredients. Stir just until the dry ingredients are moistened.
6. Pour into the prepared loaf pan.
7. Sprinkle the fresh tomato, bell pepper and mozzarella cheese over the batter.
8. Bake for 55 minutes to 1 hour or until a wooden toothpick inserted in the centre comes out clean.
9. Remove from the oven. Transfer the bread to a rack to cool.

This can be stored in an airtight container for up to 2 days or frozen for up to 2 months.

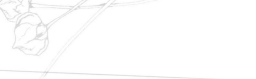

QUICK SEED BREAD

1½ cups (375 mL) unbleached
  all-purpose flour
¾ cup (175 mL) lightly packed
  brown sugar
½ cup (125 mL) whole wheat flour
½ cup (125 mL) sunflower seeds,
  lightly toasted (see sidebar)
⅓ cup (75 mL) ground flaxseed
2 Tbsp (25 mL) whole flaxseed
  (more for sprinkling)

2 Tbsp (25 mL) poppy seeds
2 Tbsp (25 mL) sesame seeds
1 tsp (5 mL) baking powder
1 tsp (5 mL) baking soda
½ tsp (2 mL) salt
1¼ cups (300 mL) buttermilk
  (see page 18)
¼ cup (50 mL) canola oil
1 large egg, beaten

Topping

1 tsp (5 mL) whole flaxseed
1 tsp (5 mL) sesame seeds

1 tsp (5 mL) raw sunflower
  seeds

YIELD: 1 loaf (16 slices)

NUTRIENT VALUES PER
SERVING (1 SLICE)

Calories	185
Protein	4.9 g
Carbohydrates	24.9 g
Fibre	2.6 g
Fat	8.4 g
Saturated	1.5 g
Monounsaturated	3.1 g
Polyunsaturated	3.5 g
Cholesterol	14 mg
Folate	32 mcg
Potassium	162 mg
Sodium	201 mg

TO TOAST SUNFLOWER
SEEDS, preheat the oven to
350°F (180°C). Place ½ cup
(125 mL) of sunflower seeds
on a pie plate. Toast for
3 minutes, stir, toast for
another 3 minutes and stir
again. Toast 2 to 3 minutes
more, until lightly browned.

1. Preheat the oven to 350°F (180°C). Spray a 9- × 5-inch (2 L) loaf pan with
   non-stick cooking spray.
2. In a large bowl, combine the all-purpose flour, brown sugar, whole wheat flour,
   sunflower seeds, ground and 2 Tbsp (25 mL) whole flaxseed, poppy seeds,
   sesame seeds, baking powder, baking soda and salt. Stir well.
3. In another bowl, beat together the buttermilk, oil and egg. Add to the dry
   ingredients. Stir until just moistened.
4. Pour the batter into the prepared loaf pan.
5. Sprinkle the 1 tsp (5 mL) whole flaxseed, sesame and sunflower seeds over
   the batter.
6. Bake for 55 to 65 minutes or until a wooden toothpick inserted in the centre
   comes out clean.
7. Remove from the oven. Cool in the pan for 10 minutes, then turn out onto
   a rack to cool completely.

*This can be stored in an airtight container for up to 2 days or frozen for up to
2 months.*

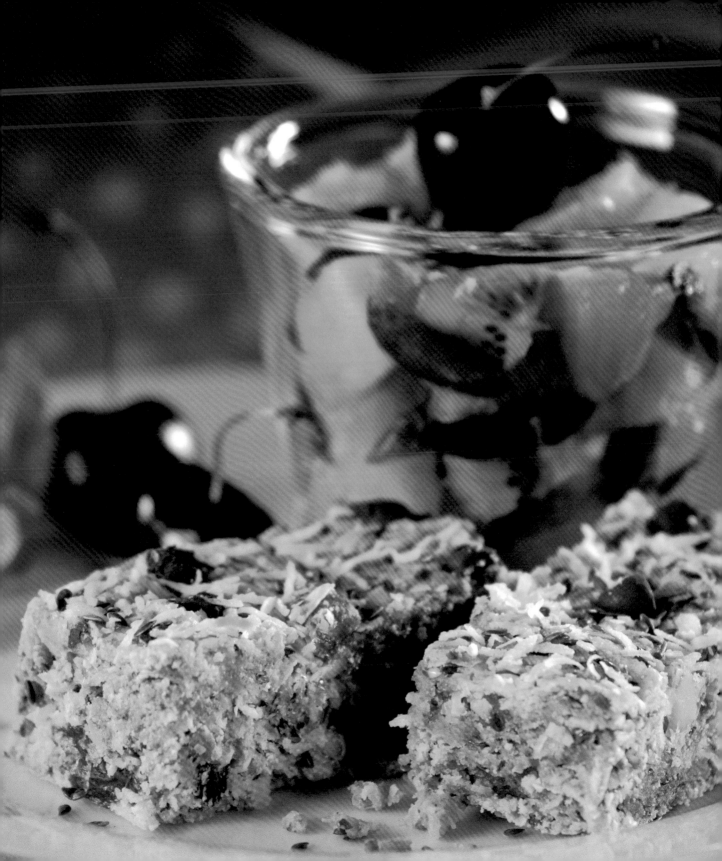

FLAX HEALTH BARS

1 cup (250 mL) lightly packed
   brown sugar

⅔ cup (150 mL) butter, softened

½ cup (125 mL) granulated sugar

1 Tbsp (15 mL) vanilla extract

2 eggs

2 cups (500 mL) unbleached
   all-purpose flour

⅓ cup (75 mL) ground toasted
   golden flaxseed

2 cups (500 mL) Special K
   (or similar) cereal

1 cup (250 mL) old-fashioned
   rolled oats

1 cup (250 mL) quick-cooking oats

½ cup (125 mL) combination of
   raisins, chocolate chips, coconut,
   chopped nuts, cran-raisins, etc.

⅓ cup (75 mL) whole toasted
   golden flaxseed

¼ cup (50 mL) raw sunflower seeds

YIELD: one 9- × 13-inch (23 ×
33 cm) baking pan (30 bars)

NUTRIENT VALUES PER
SERVING (1 BAR)

Calories	176
Protein	3.5 g
Carbohydrates	24.9 g
Fibre	1.9 g
Fat	7.4 g
Saturated	3.3 g
Monounsaturated	2.1 g
Polyunsaturated	1.5 g
Cholesterol	25 mg
Folate	23 mcg
Potassium	105 mg
Sodium	65 mg

*Based on recipe using equal
amounts of raisins, chocolate
chips, coconut, chopped pecans
and cran-raisins*

1. Preheat the oven to 350°F (180°C). Spray a 9- × 13-inch (23 × 33 cm) baking pan with non-stick cooking spray.
2. In a bowl, cream together the brown sugar, butter, granulated sugar and vanilla.
3. Continue beating, adding 1 egg at a time.
4. Add the flour and ground flaxseed. Stir until well combined.
5. Add the cereal, rolled oats, quick-cooking oats, raisin combination, whole flax-seed and sunflower seeds. Stir until uniform in texture.
6. Turn into the prepared pan.
7. Bake for 13 to 15 minutes.
8. Remove from the oven and cool on a rack in the pan before cutting into bars.

These can be stored in an airtight container for up to 2 days or frozen for up to 2 months.

MAPLE OATMEAL WITH QUINOA

3 cups (750 mL) water

½ tsp (2 mL) salt

1 cup (250 mL) old-fashioned
   rolled oats

½ cup (125 mL) quinoa

⅓ cup (75 mL) raisins

2 Tbsp (25 mL) pure maple syrup

¼ tsp (1 mL) ground cinnamon

¼ cup (50 mL) chopped walnuts or
   sliced almonds

2 Tbsp (25 mL) whole flaxseed

2 Tbsp (25 mL) ground flaxseed

YIELD: 5 servings

NUTRIENT VALUES PER
SERVING (¾ CUP/175 ML)

Calories	262
Protein	8.6 g
Carbohydrates	41.8 g
Fibre	5.7 g
Fat	9.0 g
Saturated	2.0 g
Monounsaturated	2.3 g
Polyunsaturated	4.2 g
Cholesterol	0 mg
Folate	23 mcg
Potassium	381 mg
Sodium	245 mg

Based on recipe using walnuts

QUINOA IS AN ANCIENT
GRAIN. It is tiny and bead-shaped, ivory-coloured and delicately flavoured. It contains protein and is higher in unsaturated fats and lower in carbohydrates than other grains. You can find it in health food stores and some grocery stores.

1. In a medium saucepan, bring the water to a rolling boil. Add the salt.
2. Stir in the oats, quinoa, raisins, maple syrup and cinnamon. Simmer until all the water is absorbed and the oatmeal is thick, about 18 minutes.
3. Stir in the walnuts and the whole and ground flaxseed.
4. Cover, remove from the heat and let stand for 2 minutes.

Serve with warm milk, drizzle with extra maple syrup and top with fresh blueberries if desired.

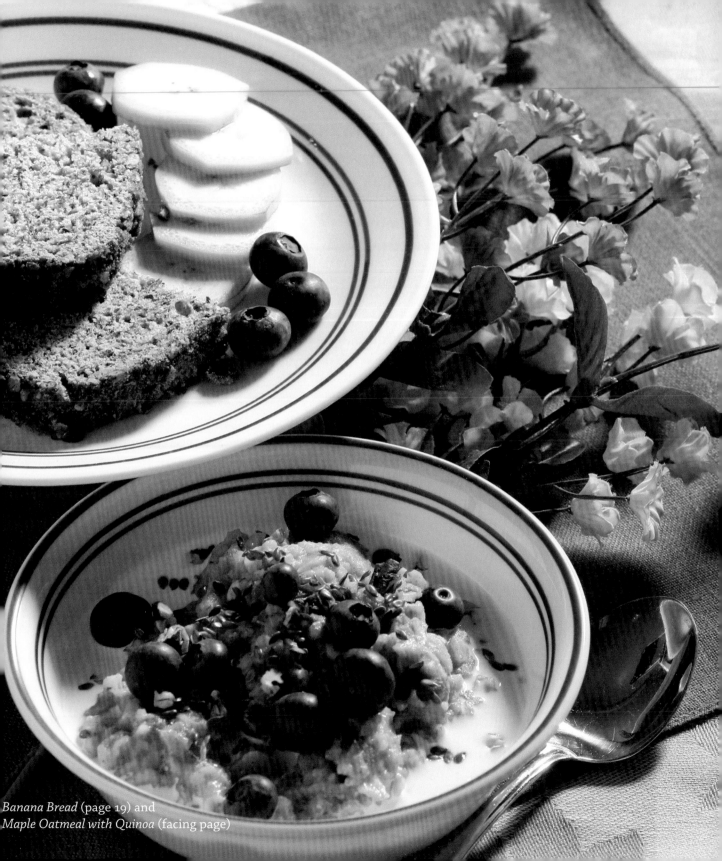

Banana Bread (page 19) and
Maple Oatmeal with Quinoa (facing page)

PROTEIN BREAKFAST SQUARES

1 cup (250 mL) spelt flakes or old-fashioned rolled oats

½ cup (125 mL) lightly packed brown sugar

½ cup (125 mL) almond butter

1 cup (250 mL) boiling water

½ cup (125 mL) plain yogurt

1 tsp (5 mL) almond extract

2 eggs, slightly beaten

½ cup (125 mL) low-fat soy flour

½ cup (125 mL) unbleached all-purpose flour

⅓ cup (75 mL) ground flaxseed

1 tsp (5 mL) baking soda

½ cup (125 mL) chopped pitted dates

½ cup (125 mL) chopped almonds

YIELD: one 9-inch (23 cm) square pan (16 squares)

NUTRIENT VALUES PER SERVING (1 SQUARE)

Calories	190
Protein	6.5 g
Carbohydrates	22.7 g
Fibre	2.6 g
Fat	9.3 g
Saturated	1.5 g
Monounsaturated	5.2 g
Polyunsaturated	2.2 g
Cholesterol	24 mg
Folate	30 mcg
Potassium	291 mg
Sodium	99 mg

1. In a large bowl, combine the spelt flakes, brown sugar and almond butter.
2. Pour the boiling water overtop, stir well and let stand for 20 minutes.
3. Preheat the oven to 350°F (180°C). Spray a 9-inch (23 cm) square pan with non-stick cooking spray.
4. Stir the yogurt, almond extract and beaten eggs into the spelt-flake mixture.
5. In a medium bowl, combine both flours, the ground flaxseed and baking soda.
6. Add to the spelt mixture along with the dates. Mix together until moistened.
7. Spread the mixture into the prepared pan.
8. Sprinkle with the chopped almonds.
9. Bake for 30 to 40 minutes or until a wooden toothpick inserted in the centre comes out clean.
10. Remove from the oven and place on a rack to cool in the pan.
11. When cool, cut into 16 squares.

These can be stored in an airtight container for up to 2 days or frozen for up to 2 months.

GRANOLA

6 cups (1.5 L) 9 Grain cereal

1 cup (250 mL) shredded unsweetened coconut

½ cup (125 mL) sliced almonds

⅓ cup (75 mL) sesame seeds

½ tsp (2 mL) salt

½ cup (125 mL) hot water
(150°F/70°C)

½ cup (125 mL) liquid honey

¼ cup (50 mL) canola oil

1½ cups (375 mL) finely chopped dried
fruit mix (peach, apple, apricot,
prune)

1 cup (250 mL) ground flaxseed

YIELD: 10 cups (2.5 L)

NUTRIENT VALUES PER
SERVING (⅓ CUP/75 ML)

Calories	164
Protein	4.8 g
Carbohydrates	26.3 g
Fibre	5.8 g
Fat	6.6 g
Saturated	1.4 g
Monounsaturated	2.2 g
Polyunsaturated	1.5 g
Cholesterol	0 mg
Folate	2 mcg
Potassium	231 mg
Sodium	44 mg

1. Preheat the oven to 325°F (160°C).
2. Mix together the 9 Grain cereal, coconut, almonds, sesame seeds and salt in a large roasting pan.
3. Mix together the hot water, honey and canola oil in a bowl.
4. Pour this over the dry mixture, mixing well until evenly moistened.
5. Bake for 1 hour, stirring every 15 minutes, until the oats are crisp and golden.
6. Remove from the oven.
7. Stir in the mixed fruit and flaxseed.
8. Cool in the roasting pan, stirring occasionally.

Serve in small bowls with cold or warmed milk or sprinkle over yogurt, fresh fruit or berries. Store in an airtight container or in plastic bags in the refrigerator or freezer.

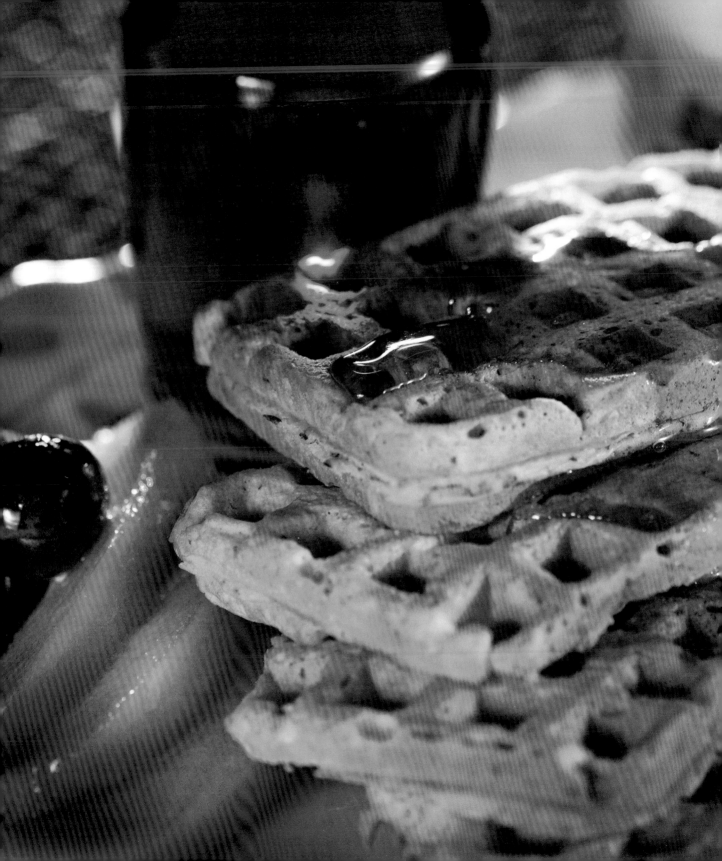

FLAX WAFFLES

1¼ cups (300 mL) unbleached
all-purpose flour

¼ cup (50 mL) ground flaxseed

1 Tbsp (15 mL) baking powder

1 Tbsp (15 mL) granulated sugar

½ tsp (2 mL) salt

2 large eggs, separated

1 cup (250 mL) 1% milk

2 Tbsp (25 mL) flaxseed oil

¼ tsp (1 mL) vanilla extract

YIELD: about 10 waffles

NUTRIENT VALUES PER
SERVING (2 WAFFLES)

Calories	253
Protein	8.6 g
Carbohydrates	31.7 g
Fibre	2.8 g
Fat	10.9 g
Saturated	2.6 g
Monounsaturated	2.7 g
Polyunsaturated	5.0 g
Cholesterol	76 mg
Folate	57 mcg
Potassium	188 mg
Sodium	442 mg

1. In a large bowl, combine the flour, ground flaxseed, baking powder, sugar and salt. Blend well.
2. In another bowl, whisk the egg yolks until thick.
3. Add the milk, flaxseed oil and vanilla to the egg yolks and mix well.
4. Combine the wet mixture with the dry ingredients. Mix until smooth.
5. Beat the egg whites in a separate bowl until soft peaks form. Fold into the batter.
6. Heat and prepare a waffle iron according to the manufacturer's directions.
7. Scoop the batter onto the waffle iron and cook until there is no more steam escaping from the sides.

Serve with maple syrup, fresh fruit, whipped cream, etc.

SWEET POTATO PANCAKES

Flax Fact: A flax plant can grow to around 16 to 36 inches (40 to 91 cm) and is self-pollinating.

2 cups (500 mL) grated sweet potato, lightly packed

2 Tbsp (25 mL) grated onion

2 Tbsp (25 mL) chopped fresh cilantro or parsley

1 large egg, slightly beaten

⅓ cup (75 mL) whole wheat flour

¼ cup (50 mL) ground flaxseed

1 tsp (5 mL) baking powder

½ tsp (2 mL) salt

½ tsp (2 mL) curry powder

¼ cup (50 mL) 1% milk

2 Tbsp (25 mL) melted butter

canola oil for frying

YIELD: 14 to 16 pancakes

NUTRIENT VALUES PER SERVING (3 PANCAKES)

Calories	160
Protein	5.1 g
Carbohydrates	22.3 g
Fibre	4.3 g
Fat	7.1 g
Saturated	2.9 g
Monounsaturated	1.8 g
Polyunsaturated	1.4 g
Cholesterol	50 mg
Folate	16 mcg
Potassium	225 mg
Sodium	361 mg

1. In a bowl, combine the sweet potato, onion, cilantro and egg.
2. Add the flour, flaxseed, baking powder, salt and curry powder. Stir.
3. Add the milk and butter. Stir to form a batter.
4. Heat a non-stick skillet over medium heat.
5. Add 1 to 2 tsp (5 to 10 mL) canola oil. Swirl to coat the pan.
6. Using a 1 Tbsp (15 mL) measure, drop a rounded scoop of batter into the skillet and flatten it slightly with the back of the spoon.
7. Cook for 1 to 1½ minutes or until the pancake is nicely browned on the bottom and around its edges.
8. Flip the pancake over, gently pressing down on it with the back of a pancake turner, and cook for 1 to 1½ minutes or until cooked through.
9. Continue cooking pancakes until all the batter is used, adding more oil to the pan as needed.

Serve with plain yogurt and mango chutney. This is a nice accompaniment for the Pan-Roasted Pork Tenderloin with Flax Crust, and they are pictured together on page 142.

APPLE PANCAKES

1¼ cups (300 mL) unbleached
all-purpose flour

⅓ cup (75 mL) ground flaxseed

3 Tbsp (45 mL) granulated sugar

1 Tbsp (15 mL) baking powder

½ tsp (2 mL) salt

¼ tsp (1 mL) ground cinnamon

pinch nutmeg

2 eggs, separated, whites beaten stiffly

1¼ cups (300 mL) 2% milk

3 Tbsp (45 mL) butter, melted

1 cup (250 mL) pared and shredded
apple (shred just prior to adding
to batter)

YIELD: about 12 pancakes

NUTRIENT VALUES PER
SERVING (2 PANCAKES)

Calories	278
Protein	8.2 g
Carbohydrates	36.0 g
Fibre	2.8 g
Fat	11.7 g
Saturated	2.5 g
Monounsaturated	3.8 g
Polyunsaturated	4.6 g
Cholesterol	75 mg
Folate	44 mcg
Potassium	266 mg
Sodium	472 mg

1. In a large bowl, combine the flour, flaxseed, sugar, baking powder, salt, cinnamon and nutmeg.
2. In a medium bowl, lightly beat together the egg yolks, milk and butter.
3. Add to the dry ingredients and stir until just combined.
4. Shred the apple, add it to the batter and stir until just combined.
5. Fold in the egg whites.
6. Preheat a griddle or heavy skillet to medium heat. Spray with non-stick cooking spray.
7. Measure ⅓ cup (75 mL) of batter into the hot pan for each pancake.
8. Cook the pancakes until bubbles appear on the surface, about 1 minute.
9. Turn over and brown the other side.

Serve with maple syrup, applesauce, whipped cream, etc.

CREAMY MANGO SMOOTHIE

YIELD: 2 servings

NUTRIENT VALUES PER
SERVING (1½ CUPS/
375 ML)

Calories	298
Protein	5.5 g
Carbohydrates	46.4 g
Fibre	2.1 g
Fat	11.6 g
Saturated	1.7 g
Monounsaturated	2.0 g
Polyunsaturated	6.3 g
Cholesterol	5 mg
Folate	21 mcg
Potassium	362 mg
Sodium	165 mg

1 cup (250 mL) peach mango–
flavoured tofu

1 cup (250 mL) 1% milk

1 large ripe mango, peeled
and pitted

4 tsp (20 mL) flaxseed oil

1. Put the tofu, milk, mango and flaxseed oil in a blender.
2. Blend until smooth, about 45 seconds.
3. Pour into 2 tall glasses.

THICK BERRY SMOOTHIE

YIELD: 2 servings

NUTRIENT VALUES PER
SERVING (1½ CUPS/
375 ML)

Calories	321
Protein	7.9 g
Carbohydrates	71.2 g
Fibre	7.6 g
Fat	3.9 g
Saturated	1.5 g
Monounsaturated	1.0 g
Polyunsaturated	1.1 g
Cholesterol	0 mg
Folate	42 mcg
Potassium	538 mg
Sodium	53 mg

*Based on recipe using equal
parts frozen raspberries,
strawberries and blueberries*

1½ cups (375 mL) fat-free plain
soy milk

½ cup (125 mL) unsweetened
orange juice

1 frozen banana, peeled

1 cup (250 mL) frozen mixed berries

2 Tbsp (25 mL) ground flaxseed

2 Tbsp (25 mL) concentrated blackcurrant nectar (optional)

1. Pour the soy milk and orange juice into a blender.
2. Cut or break the banana in half. Add it to the soy mixture.
3. Add the berries, flaxseed and blackcurrant nectar (if using).
4. Blend until thick and smooth, about 45 seconds.
5. Pour into 2 tall glasses.

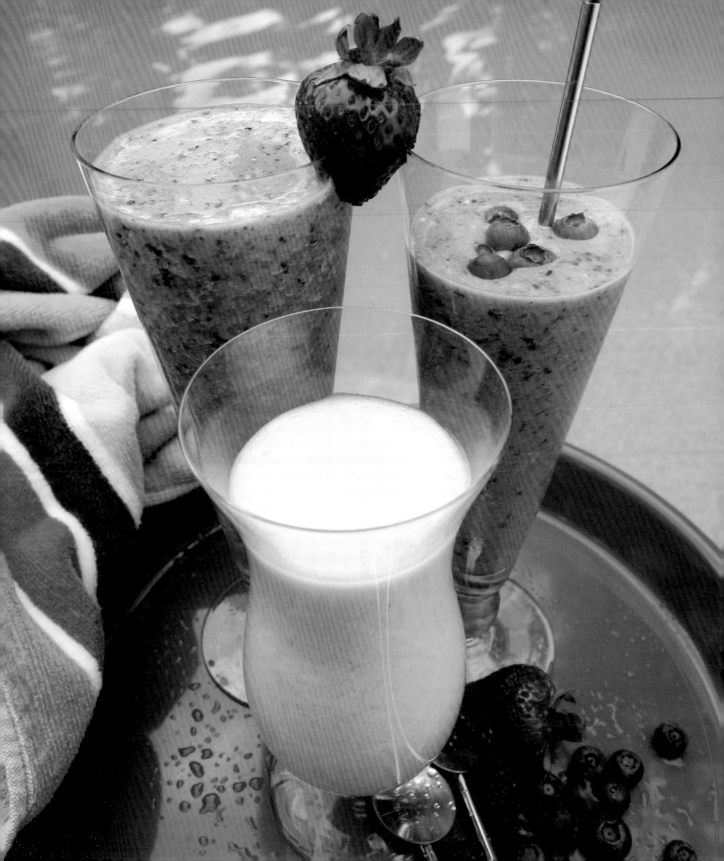

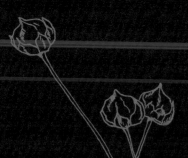
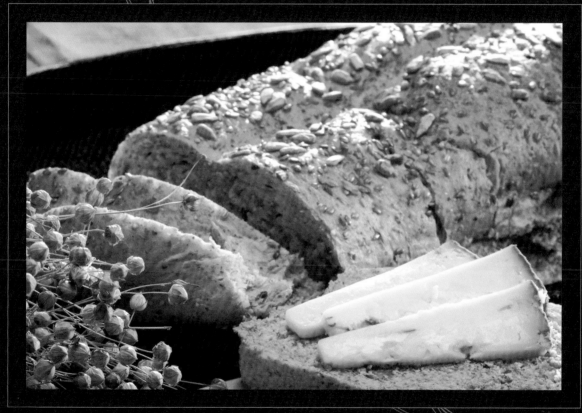
Pictured: *Grain Bread* (page 48)
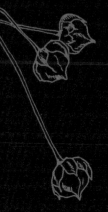

Breads, Buns & More

Many people recognize flax most easily as a bakery ingredient. It appears as an integral component of multi-grain breads and as a topping for bagels and specialty breads.

Flax allows the home baker to bring an old-world food into a new-world kitchen! In its whole form, flax is extremely stable, making it readily available for bread-baking sessions.

Tortillas and pitas, also some of the earliest breads known to man, have strong roots in many cultures. No matter their shape, baked grain products passed from generation to generation are immensely satisfying.

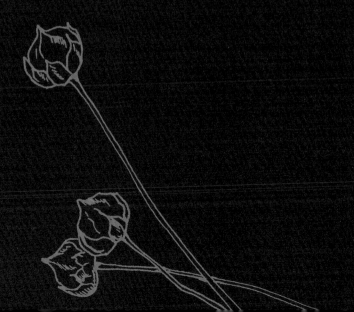

CLASSIC FLAX BREAD

7 cups (1.75 L) unbleached
   all-purpose flour

1 cup (250 mL) ground flaxseed

¼ cup (50 mL) granulated sugar

1 Tbsp (15 mL) quick-rising yeast

2 tsp (10 mL) salt

2 cups (500 mL) water

1 cup (250 mL) skim milk

1 Tbsp (15 mL) shortening

YIELD: 2 loaves (16 slices per loaf)

NUTRIENT VALUES PER SERVING (1 SLICE)

Calories	131
Protein	4.1 g
Carbohydrates	24.3 g
Fibre	2.1 g
Fat	2.4 g
Saturated	0.9 g
Monounsaturated	0.7 g
Polyunsaturated	0.7 g
Cholesterol	0 mg
Folate	57 mcg
Potassium	79 mg
Sodium	153 mg

1. Reserve 1 cup (250 mL) of the flour. Mix the remaining flour with the flaxseed, sugar, yeast and salt in a large bowl.

2. Heat the water, milk and shortening in a saucepan over medium heat (or in a glass bowl in the microwave) until hot to the touch, 120 to 130°F (50 to 55°C). Stir the hot liquids into the flour-flaxseed mixture. Gradually mix in enough of the reserved flour to make a soft dough that doesn't stick to the bowl.

3. Turn the dough out onto a floured board and knead until smooth and elastic, about 8 minutes. Cover the dough and let it rest for 10 minutes.

4. Preheat the oven to 400°F (200°C). Spray two 8½- × 4½-inch (1.5 L) loaf pans with non-stick cooking spray.

5. Divide the dough into 2 equal portions and turn into the prepared pans.

6. Bake the bread for 30 to 35 minutes. Remove from the pans and cool on a rack.

This can be stored in an airtight container for up to 2 days or frozen for up to 2 months.

GRAIN BREAD

Flax Fact: In the fifth century, Hippocrates extolled the healing properties of flax.

1 cup + 3½ cups (250 mL + 875 mL) hot water (150°F/70°C), divided

½ cup (125 mL) liquid honey

three 8 g packages active dry yeast (3 Tbsp/45 mL)

¾ cup (175 mL) skim milk powder

⅓ cup (75 mL) canola oil

1 Tbsp (15 mL) salt

5 cups (1.25 L) whole wheat flour

5 cups (1.25 L) unbleached all-purpose flour

1½ cups (375 mL) ground flaxseed

¾ cup (175 mL) cracked wheat

¾ cup + 3 Tbsp (175 mL + 45 mL) raw sunflower seeds, divided

¼ cup + 2 Tbsp (50 mL + 30 mL) whole flaxseed, divided

¼ cup (50 mL) millet

2 eggs, beaten

cornmeal or unbleached all-purpose flour

1 egg white

1 Tbsp (15 mL) water

YIELD: 3 loaves (16 slices per loaf)

NUTRIENT VALUES PER SERVING (1 SLICE)

Calories	160
Protein	5.7 g
Carbohydrates	26.5 g
Fibre	3.9 g
Fat	4.7 g
Saturated	1.2 g
Monounsaturated	2.9 g
Polyunsaturated	10.0 g
Cholesterol	0 mg
Folate	69 mcg
Potassium	210 mg
Sodium	1 mg

1. In a medium bowl, combine 1 cup (250 mL) of the hot water with the honey. Stir and let stand until the water reaches 100 to 110°F (40 to 45°C), about 7 minutes.
2. Sprinkle the yeast overtop and let stand for 15 minutes.
3. In a large bread-mixing bowl, combine the remaining 3½ cups (875 mL) of hot water with the skim milk powder, oil and salt. Cool for 15 minutes.
4. In another large bowl, combine both flours, the ground flaxseed, cracked wheat, ¾ cup (175 mL) sunflower seeds, ¼ cup (50 mL) whole flaxseed and millet.
5. Stir the yeast mixture and beaten eggs into the milk mixture.
6. Gradually add 4 cups (1 L) of the flour mixture to the liquid mixture. Mix well.
7. Add all of the remaining flour mixture while continuing to mix.
8. Turn the dough onto a clean, floured work surface, gradually adding up to ½ cup (125 mL) more unbleached flour to make a medium-soft dough.
9. Rub canola oil on your hands and knead the dough until smooth and elastic in texture, about 8 to 10 minutes.
10. Place the dough in an oiled bowl, oil the top of the dough and cover loosely with plastic wrap.
11. Let rise in a warm place for 1 hour.
12. Punch the dough down, then let it rise for another half hour.

13. Sprinkle a 12- × 18-inch (30 × 45 cm) baking sheet with cornmeal or flour.

14. Divide the dough into 3 equal portions. Shape each portion into a 3- × 11-inch (8 × 28 cm) log-shaped loaf. Place the loaves evenly spaced apart on the prepared baking sheet.

15. In a bowl, beat together the egg white and water until frothy. Brush the tops of the loaves.

16. Sprinkle 1 Tbsp (15 mL) of sunflower seeds and 2 tsp (10 mL) of whole flaxseed over each loaf.

17. Cover and let rise until doubled in size, about 45 minutes.

18. Preheat the oven to 350°F (180°C).

19. Bake for 30 to 40 minutes or until the loaves are nicely browned and make a hollow sound when their tops are tapped.

20. Remove from the oven and let cool for 5 minutes.

21. Remove from the pan and continue cooling on a rack.

Store well-wrapped in plastic for up to 2 days or frozen for up to 2 months. Pictured on page 102.

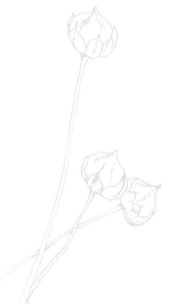

BARLEY & FLAX BEER BREAD

1½ cups (375 mL) unbleached
   all-purpose flour
¾ cup (175 mL) barley flour
½ cup (125 mL) ground flaxseed
1 Tbsp (15 mL) baking powder
1 tsp (5 mL) baking soda

½ tsp (2 mL) salt
1 large egg
2 Tbsp (25 mL) liquid honey
12 fl oz (341 mL) bottle or 13 fl oz
   (355 mL) can beer (see sidebar)

YIELD: 1 loaf (16 slices)

NUTRIENT VALUES PER
SERVING (1 SLICE)

Calories	94
Protein	3.1 g
Carbohydrates	16.2 g
Fibre	2.1 g
Fat	2.2 g
Saturated	0.8 g
Monounsaturated	0.6 g
Polyunsaturated	0.6 g
Cholesterol	13 mg
Folate	19 mcg
Potassium	66 mg
Sodium	239 mg

USE DE-ALCOHOLIZED
BEER if you prefer.

1. Preheat the oven to 350°F (180°C). Spray a 4½- × 8½-inch (1.5 L) loaf pan with non-stick cooking spray.

2. In a bowl, combine both flours, the ground flaxseed, baking powder, baking soda and salt. Stir well.

3. In another bowl, use a fork to beat together the egg and honey. Gently stir in the beer.

4. Add the liquid ingredients to the dry ingredients and mix just until moistened.

5. Spoon into the prepared loaf pan.

6. Bake for 40 to 50 minutes or until a wooden toothpick inserted in the centre comes out clean.

7. Remove from the oven and transfer to a rack to cool.

This is best eaten the same day, but it's also tasty when toasted the next day.

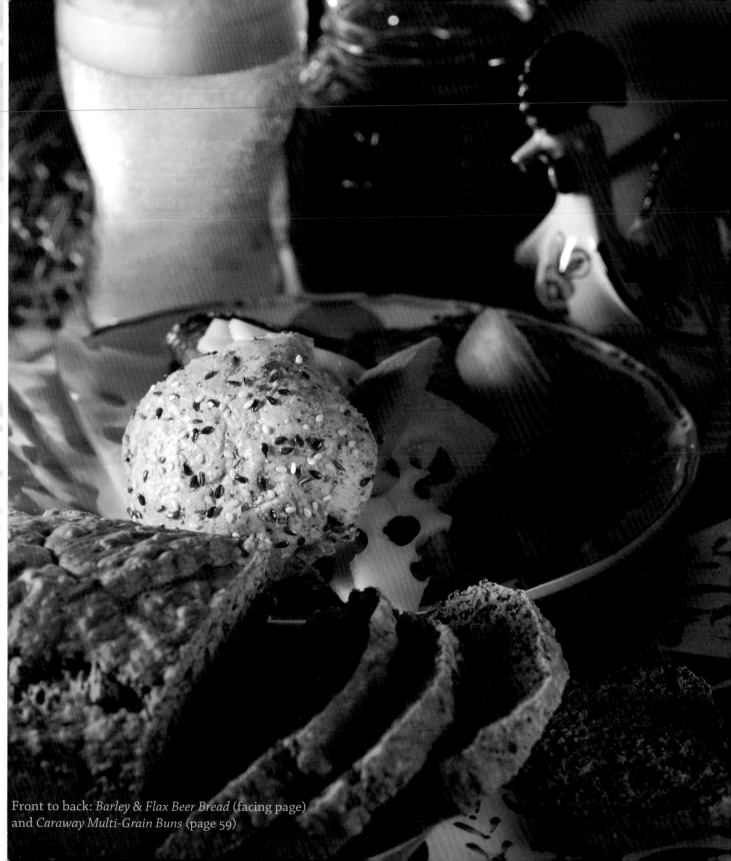

Front to back: *Barley & Flax Beer Bread* (facing page)
and *Caraway Multi-Grain Buns* (page 59)

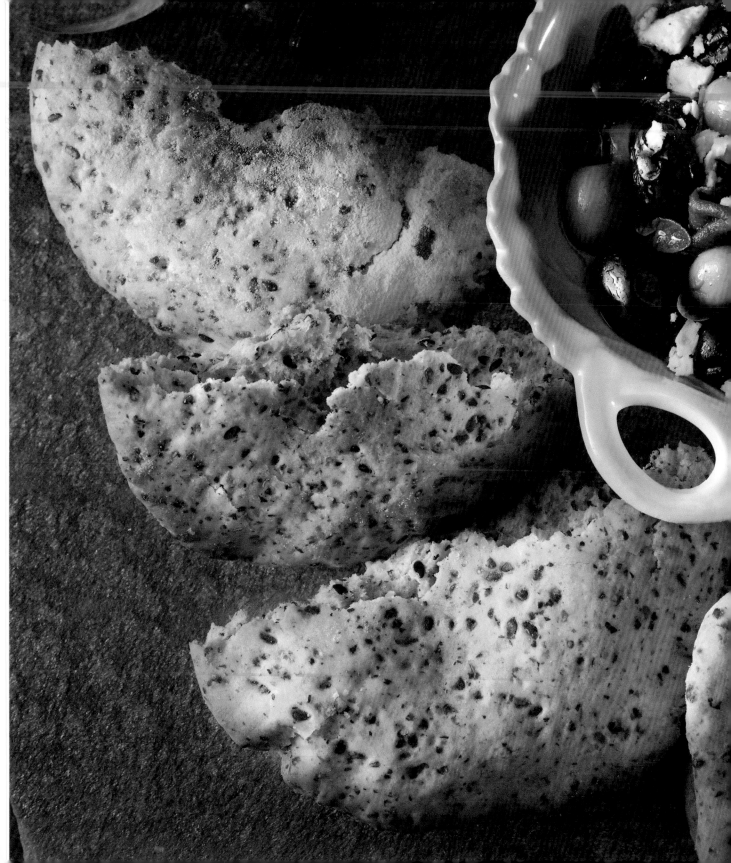

HERB & GARLIC PITA

2½ cups (625 mL) unbleached
   all-purpose flour
one 8 g package active dry yeast
   (2¼ tsp/11 mL)
1 tsp (5 mL) granulated sugar
½ tsp (2 mL) salt
1 cup (250 mL) warm water (100 to
   110°F/40 to 45°C)

¼ cup (50 mL) ground flaxseed
2 tsp (10 mL) whole flaxseed
2 tsp (10 mL) crushed dried basil
2 tsp (10 mL) crushed dried oregano
½ tsp (2 mL) garlic powder
1 Tbsp (15 mL) flaxseed oil

YIELD: 6 pitas

NUTRIENT VALUES PER
SERVING (1 WHOLE PITA)

Calories	230
Protein	7.1 g
Carbohydrates	40.4 g
Fibre	3.2 g
Fat	4.8 g
Saturated	1.2 g
Monounsaturated	1.1 g
Polyunsaturated	2.3 g
Cholesterol	0 mg
Folate	102 mcg
Potassium	76 mg
Sodium	163 mg

1. In the bowl of a stand mixer, combine 1 cup (250 mL) of the flour with the yeast, sugar and salt.
2. Add the water and beat for 2 minutes on medium speed.
3. Add ½ cup (125 mL) of the flour, the ground and whole flaxseed, basil, oregano and garlic powder. Beat on high for 1 minute.
4. Gradually add the remaining flour to make a soft dough.
5. Knead the dough on a clean, floured work surface until smooth, about 5 to 7 minutes.
6. Place the dough in a large oiled bowl. Turn the dough to oil all sides. Cover.
7. Set in a warm spot to rise until doubled in bulk, about 1 hour.
8. Punch down the dough and let rest for another ½ hour.
9. Preheat the oven to 450°F (230°C). Lightly flour 2 baking sheets.
10. Divide the dough into 6 equal pieces. Shape each piece into a ball.
11. On a clean, floured work surface, form a pita by rolling each ball into a flat 6-inch (15 cm) circle. Place the pitas on the prepared baking sheets.
12. Bake in the centre of the oven until the pitas are puffed and brown, about 15 minutes. Remove to a clean work surface.
13. Brush the tops lightly with flaxseed oil.
14. Let cool for 5 minutes. Put the pitas in a large plastic bag but do not seal until completely cool.

These can be stored in an airtight container for up to 2 days or frozen for up to 2 months.

Continued on the next page . . .

Serving Suggestions

Pita Chips *(Yield: 2 servings)*

1. Preheat the oven to 325°F (160°C).
2. Split the pita in half into 2 rounds.
3. Cut each round into 8 wedges for 16 wedges in total.
4. Lay them flat on a baking sheet.
5. Bake until dry, about 5 to 6 minutes.
6. Serve with hummus, baba ghanouj or your favourite dip.

Greek Salad Pita

1 tomato, diced	½ tsp (2 mL) crushed dried oregano
⅓ cup (75 mL) diced cucumber	1 pita, halved crosswise
2 Tbsp (25 mL) diced red onion	ranch dressing
¼ cup (50 mL) crumbled feta cheese	

1. In a bowl, toss together the tomato, cucumber, onion, feta and oregano.
2. Open the pita on its cut side to form a pocket.
3. Divide the filling mixture between both pockets.
4. Drizzle with ranch dressing.

Pita Pizza

1. Use a whole pita shell as a pizza base.
2. Top with pizza sauce, topping and cheese of your choice.
3. Heat in the centre of a preheated 400°F (200°C) oven until the cheese melts.

CARAWAY MULTI-GRAIN BUNS

two 8 g packages active dry yeast
  (5 tsp/25 mL)

3 cups (750 mL) warm water (100 to
  110°F/40 to 45°C)

⅓ cup (75 mL) canola oil

2 Tbsp (25 mL) fancy molasses

2 tsp (10 mL) caraway seeds (more
  for sprinkling)

1½ tsp (7 mL) salt

½ tsp (2 mL) white vinegar

1 large egg, beaten

1 cup (250 mL) whole wheat flour

1 cup (250 mL) oat bran

1 cup (250 mL) rye flour

1 cup (250 mL) ground flaxseed

¼ cup (50 mL) whole flaxseed

¼ cup (50 mL) sesame seeds

¼ cup (50 mL) raw sunflower seeds

3½ to 4 cups (875 mL to 1 L) unbleached
  all-purpose flour

1 egg white

1 Tbsp (15 mL) water

2 Tbsp (25 mL) whole flaxseed

1 Tbsp (15 mL) caraway seeds

1 Tbsp (15 mL) sesame seeds

YIELD: 24 buns

NUTRIENT VALUES PER
SERVING (1 BUN)

Calories	200
Protein	7.0 g
Carbohydrates	28.4 g
Fibre	5.3 g
Fat	8.6 g
Saturated	2.0 g
Monounsaturated	3.4 g
Polyunsaturated	2.9 g
Cholesterol	9 mg
Folate	37 mcg
Potassium	177 mg
Sodium	151 mg

ACTIVE DRY YEAST is a form of baker's yeast and is available as regular and quick-rising. It's alive but remains dormant until moisture is added.

1. In a large bowl, dissolve the yeast in the warm water.
2. Add the oil, molasses, caraway seeds, salt, vinegar and egg. Stir.
3. Add the whole wheat flour, oat bran, rye flour, ground flaxseed, whole flaxseed and sesame and sunflower seeds. Beat until smooth.
4. Gradually add enough all-purpose flour to form a soft dough. Turn it out onto a clean, floured work surface and knead until smooth, about 6 to 8 minutes.
5. Place in an oiled bowl, turning once to oil the top. Cover and let rise in a warm place until doubled in bulk, about 1 hour.
6. Spray a baking sheet with non-stick cooking spray.
7. Punch the dough down. Shape the dough into 24 round balls and flatten each into a 3-inch (8 cm) circle.
8. Place the buns on the prepared baking sheet 2 inches (5 cm) apart.
9. Beat the egg white with the 1 Tbsp (15 mL) of water until frothy. Brush over the buns. Sprinkle the whole flaxseed, caraway and sesame seeds on the buns.
10. Cover the buns with the oiled plastic wrap. Let rise until they double in bulk, about 50 minutes. Preheat the oven to 375°F (190°C).
11. Bake for 22 to 24 minutes, until golden brown.

These can be stored in an airtight container for up to 2 days or frozen for up to 2 months. Pictured on page 51.

FLAX BUNS

2 cups (500 mL) hot water
  (150°F/70°C)

1 cup (250 mL) milk

½ cup (125 mL) melted margarine

½ cup (125 mL) granulated sugar

1 Tbsp (15 mL) white vinegar

2 tsp (10 mL) salt

2 eggs

½ cup (125 mL) ground flaxseed

1 Tbsp (15 mL) quick-rising yeast

7 to 9 cups (1.75 to 2.25 L) whole
  wheat flour

3 cups (750 mL) unbleached
  all-purpose flour

YIELD: 4 dozen buns

NUTRIENT VALUES PER
SERVING (1 BUN)

Calories	124
Protein	4.0 g
Carbohydrates	21.5 g
Fibre	2.9 g
Fat	3.1 g
Saturated	0.6 g
Monounsaturated	1.1 g
Polyunsaturated	1.1 g
Cholesterol	8 mg
Folate	28 mcg
Potassium	107 mg
Sodium	130 mg

1. In a bowl, combine the hot water, milk, margarine, sugar, vinegar, salt and eggs. Mix well.
2. Add the flaxseed and yeast.
3. Add both flours. Mix and knead until smooth.
4. Cover with a clean towel and let stand for 1 hour.
5. Spray 2 baking sheets with non-stick cooking spray.
6. Punch down the dough and form it into 48 buns. Place the buns on the prepared baking sheets.
7. Cover with a clean towel and let rise for 1 hour.
8. Preheat the oven to 400°F (200°C).
9. Bake for 15 to 20 minutes. Remove the buns from the oven and transfer to a rack to cool completely.

These can be stored in an airtight container for up to 2 days or frozen for up to 2 months.

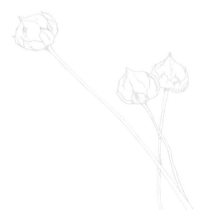

TWO-HOUR BUNS

8 cups (2 L) unbleached
   all-purpose flour

¾ cup (175 mL) ground flaxseed

2 Tbsp (25 mL) quick-rising yeast

2 eggs

½ cup (125 mL) granulated sugar

1 tsp (5 mL) salt

3 cups (750 mL) warm water
   (100 to 110°F/40 to 45°C)

YIELD: 4 dozen buns

NUTRIENT VALUES PER
SERVING (1 BUN)

Calories	109
Protein	3.3 g
Carbohydrates	20.3 g
Fibre	1.2 g
Fat	1.5 g
Saturated	0.2 g
Monounsaturated	0.3 g
Polyunsaturated	0.8 g
Cholesterol	9 mg
Folate	N/A
Potassium	74 mg
Sodium	55 mg

1. In a bowl, mix 4 cups (1 L) of the flour with the ground flaxseed and yeast.
2. In a large bowl, beat the eggs, sugar and salt. Add the water and stir.
3. Add the flour mixture to the liquid ingredients and beat with a whisk or an electric handheld mixer until well blended.
4. Add the remaining flour and knead until smooth.
5. Cover the dough with a bowl or clean towel and let it rise on the counter for 15 minutes.
6. Punch down the dough and let it rise again for 15 minutes.
7. Lightly spray 2 baking sheets with non-stick cooking spray.
8. Punch down the dough and form it into 48 buns.
9. Place the buns on the prepared baking sheets, leaving 2 inches (5 cm) between them, and cover with a clean towel.
10. Let rise for 1 hour.
11. Preheat the oven to 350°F (180°C).
12. Bake for 20 minutes. Remove the buns from the oven and transfer to a rack to cool.

These can be stored in an airtight container for up to 4 days or frozen for up to 3 months.

ONION & OLIVE FOCACCIA

Flax Fact: Flax is good for your pets, too, and is found in some pet foods.

Bread

1 cup (250 mL) warm water (100 to 110°F/40 to 45°C)
1 tsp (5 mL) granulated sugar
one 8 g package (2¼ tsp/11 mL) quick-rising yeast
2 cups (500 mL) unbleached all-purpose flour
½ cup (125 mL) ground flaxseed
1 Tbsp (15 mL) whole flaxseed
1 tsp (5 mL) salt
2 Tbsp (25 mL) canola oil
1 Tbsp (15 mL) cornmeal

Topping

2 Tbsp (25 mL) canola oil
freshly ground black pepper
¼ cup (50 mL) slivered red onion
¼ cup (50 mL) sliced black or stuffed manzanillo olives
2 Tbsp (25 mL) finely chopped fresh basil
1 Tbsp (15 mL) grated Parmesan cheese
1 tsp (5 mL) whole flaxseed

YIELD: 1 loaf (8 servings)

NUTRIENT VALUES PER SERVING (1 WEDGE)

Calories	240
Protein	6.4 g
Carbohydrates	31.2 g
Fibre	4.2 g
Fat	11.6 g
Saturated	2.4 g
Monounsaturated	4.8 g
Polyunsaturated	3.2 g
Cholesterol	1 mg
Folate	76 mcg
Potassium	144 mg
Sodium	348 mg

1. For the bread, in a bowl, combine the water and sugar. Stir well.
2. Add the yeast. Stir to dissolve.
3. In another large bowl, combine the flour, ground and whole flaxseed and salt. Mix well.
4. Add the yeast mixture and canola oil. Mix well to make a soft dough.
5. Knead the dough on a clean, floured work surface until smooth and no longer sticky, about 4 minutes.
6. Place the dough in a well-oiled bowl, turning it over to oil it evenly.
7. Cover loosely with plastic wrap. Let the dough rise in a warm place until doubled in size, about 30 to 45 minutes.
8. Spray a baking sheet or pizza pan with non-stick cooking spray. Sprinkle the pan with cornmeal.
9. Punch the dough down and form it into a ball. Press with your fingers to form a thick 10-inch (25 cm) circle.

Continued on page 64 . . .

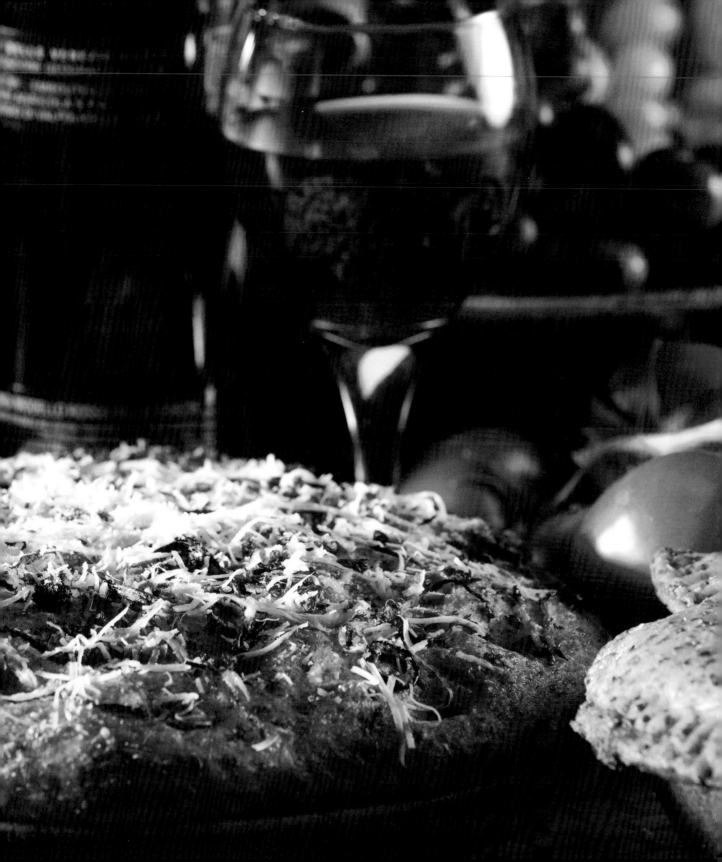

10. Place the dough on the prepared pan and cover loosely with plastic wrap. Let it rise until doubled in bulk, about half an hour.

11. Place the oven rack on the second rung from the bottom. Preheat the oven to 400°F (200°C).

12. For the topping, use your fingers to make deep depressions in the dough, about 2 inches (5 cm) apart. Drizzle canola oil overtop and season with pepper.

13. Sprinkle the onion, olives, basil, Parmesan and whole flaxseed overtop. Bake until lightly browned, about 20 to 25 minutes.

14. Cut into 8 wedges and serve warm.

This can be stored in an airtight container for up to 2 days or frozen for up to 2 months.

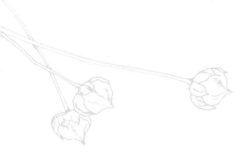

SOFT PRETZELS

2 to 3 cups (500 to 750 mL)
   unbleached all-purpose flour

2 Tbsp (25 mL) granulated sugar

1 tsp (5 mL) salt

1 Tbsp (15 mL) active dry yeast

1 cup (250 mL) water

1 Tbsp (15 mL) butter or margarine

¼ cup (50 mL) whole flaxseed

1 egg yolk

1 Tbsp (15 mL) water

coarse salt (optional)

whole flaxseed (optional)

YIELD: 12 pretzels

NUTRIENT VALUES PER
SERVING (1 PRETZEL)

Calories	162
Protein	4.7 g
Carbohydrates	28.8 g
Fibre	1.8 g
Fat	3.0 g
Saturated	0.5 g
Monounsaturated	0.9 g
Polyunsaturated	1.4 g
Cholesterol	18 mg
Folate	46 mcg
Potassium	107 mg
Sodium	214 mg

1. In a large bowl, combine 1 cup (250 mL) of the flour with the sugar, salt and yeast.
2. In a saucepan over medium-high heat, warm the water and butter to 120 to 130°F (50 to 55°C).
3. Add the warm liquid to the yeast mixture and beat until well combined. Stir in the flaxseed and gradually add enough flour to make a soft dough.
4. Turn out onto a clean, lightly floured work surface. Knead, adding more flour as necessary, until the dough is smooth and no longer sticky, about 4 minutes.
5. Place the dough in a well-oiled bowl and cover loosely with well-oiled plastic wrap. Let rise in a warm place until doubled, about 45 minutes to 1 hour.
6. Preheat the oven to 375°F (190°C). Line a baking sheet with aluminum foil and oil it lightly.
7. Punch the dough down and knead it about 5 times.
8. Divide the dough into 12 equal portions. Cover the portions you are not working on with a clean towel.
9. Roll each portion into a 16-inch (40 cm) rope and shape into a pretzel.
10. Place the pretzels on the prepared baking sheet, cover with a clean towel and let rise on the counter for 5 minutes.
11. Beat together the egg yolk and water. Lightly brush over the pretzels.
12. Sprinkle the pretzels lightly with the coarse salt and flaxseed, if using.
13. Bake for 15 minutes or until golden brown.
14. Serve with mustard or melted cream cheese for dipping.

These can be stored in an airtight container for up to 2 days or frozen for up to 2 months.

TORTILLAS

½ cup (125 mL) unbleached
  all-purpose flour
⅓ cup (75 mL) whole wheat flour
¼ cup (50 mL) ground flaxseed
1 Tbsp (15 mL) whole flaxseed

½ tsp (2 mL) salt
⅓ cup (75 mL) warm water
  (100 to 110°F/40 to 45°C)
1 tsp (5 mL) flaxseed oil

YIELD: 6 tortillas

NUTRIENT VALUES PER
SERVING (1 TORTILLA,
NO FILLING)

Calories	92
Protein	3.3 g
Carbohydrates	14.2 g
Fibre	2.8 g
Fat	3.6 g
Saturated	1.2 g
Monounsaturated	0.9 g
Polyunsaturated	1.4 g
Cholesterol	0 mg
Folate	17 mcg
Potassium	74 mg
Sodium	162 mg

1. In a medium bowl, combine both the flours, the ground and whole flaxseed and the salt.
2. In another bowl, combine the warm water and flaxseed oil.
3. Stir this into the flour mixture, adding more water 1 Tbsp (15 mL) at a time if needed to form a soft dough.
4. Knead 12 times.
5. Divide the dough into 6 equal pieces.
6. Oil your hands and shape each piece of dough into a ball. Cover with a clean towel.
7. Let rest on the counter for 15 minutes.
8. Heat a 10-inch (25 cm) cast iron skillet over medium-high heat.
9. Flatten each ball into a round patty.
10. Roll each patty out on a clean, lightly floured work surface until very thin, about 6 to 7 inches (15 to 18 cm) in diameter.
11. Cook each side for 30 to 45 seconds, until blistered and lightly browned. Do not overcook.
12. Stack the tortillas and cover them with a kitchen towel to keep them warm until you're ready to use them.

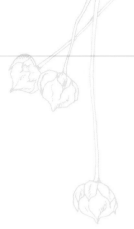

Serving Suggestions

Cheese Quesadilla

1. Sprinkle a tortilla with ¼ cup (50 mL) grated cheddar or Monterey Jack cheese.
2. Add 2 Tbsp (25 mL) chopped red onion.
3. Fold the tortilla in half and press it down with the palm of your hand.
4. Heat the skillet over medium-low heat.
5. Heat the tortilla on both sides until the cheese melts, about 1½ minutes on each side.
6. Serve with sour cream and/or salsa.

Chicken Wrap

1. Thinly slice 1 chicken breast per serving.
2. Mince 1 clove of garlic.
3. Heat a non-stick skillet over medium heat.
4. Add ½ tsp (2 mL) flaxseed oil to the skillet and sauté the chicken and garlic until cooked through, about 5 minutes.
5. Add 1 Tbsp (15 mL) salsa and 2 tsp (10 mL) sour cream.
6. Stir until heated through. Spoon the filling into a tortilla. Wrap the tortilla around the filling.

Breakfast Wrap

½ tsp (2 mL) butter	black pepper
1 large egg	1 Tbsp (15 mL) minced ham
1 Tbsp (15 mL) 1% milk	1 Tbsp (15 mL) chopped red bell pepper
salt	1 Tbsp (15 mL) chopped green onion

1. In a small non-stick skillet, melt the butter over medium heat until bubbly.
2. Add the egg and milk and season with salt and pepper. Stir well.
3. Sprinkle the ham, red bell pepper and green onion overtop.
4. Reduce the heat to low.
5. Cook, stirring occasionally, until the egg is just set, about 1½ minutes.
6. Lay the egg mixture on top of the tortilla and wrap the tortilla around the filling.
7. Serve with chilli sauce or salsa.

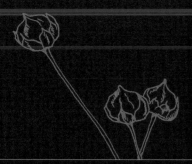

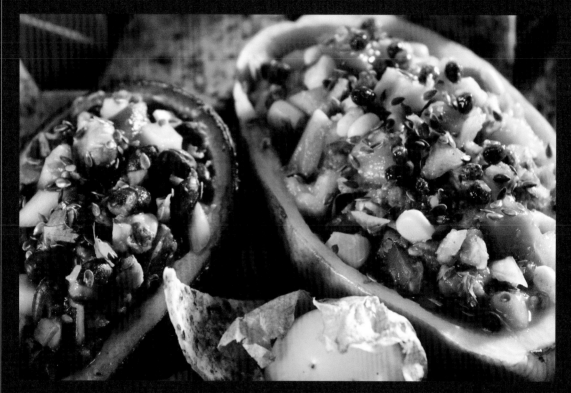

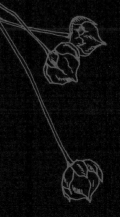

Pictured: *Summertime Salsa* and *Fiesta Salsa* (both on page 85)

Appetizers, Dips & Snacks

Once thought of as any small bite-sized food served before dinner to whet and excite the palate, today's appetizers encompass a broad range of crowd-pleasers and entertaining styles.

Cheeseballs and crackers are a mainstay of easy entertaining, as they can be made ahead and simply set out for guests to serve themselves. Dips are among the easiest and quickest appetizers to prepare. These savoury mixtures use everyday, on-hand ingredients to create an imaginative array of tastes. Salsas are a colourful fusion of flavours, textures and tastes designed for year-round appeal.

Snacks are those simple little meals that can be eaten any time of the day or night. However, they shouldn't be dismissed as "extras." Snacks are an important consideration in overall daily consumption for all age groups. For preschoolers to adolescents, wholesome snacking provides energy and essential nutrients required for growth and development.

Flaxseed, with its protein, omega-3 fatty acids, lignans and fibre, and vitamins and minerals is an ideal addition to many snack foods and hot and cold appetizers.

ANCIENT GRAIN CRACKERS

Flax Fact: By around 8000 BC the ancient Egyptians were using flax for its healing properties and keeping it as part of their medical supplies.

1 cup (250 mL) whole wheat flour

½ cup (125 mL) unbleached all-purpose flour

½ cup (125 mL) ground flaxseed

½ cup (125 mL) quinoa flour

¼ cup (50 mL) spelt flour

¼ cup (50 mL) millet flour

2 Tbsp (25 mL) whole flaxseed

1 tsp (5 mL) baking powder

½ tsp (2 mL) baking soda

½ tsp (2 mL) salt

¼ cup (50 mL) canola oil

¾ cup (175 mL) 1% milk

2 Tbsp (25 mL) brown sugar

2 Tbsp (25 mL) liquid honey

YIELD: 5 dozen crackers

NUTRIENT VALUES PER SERVING (2 CRACKERS)

Calories	78
Protein	2.2 g
Carbohydrates	11.5 g
Fibre	1.8 g
Fat	3.4 g
Saturated	0.7 g
Monounsaturated	1.5 g
Polyunsaturated	1.0 g
Cholesterol	0 mg
Folate	7 mcg
Potassium	85 mg
Sodium	74 mg

1. Preheat the oven to 350°F (180°C).
2. In a large bowl, combine the whole wheat flour, all-purpose flour, ground flaxseed, quinoa flour, spelt flour, millet flour, whole flaxseed, baking powder, baking soda and salt. Mix well.
3. Drizzle the oil over the flour mixture. Stir well, then rub it between your fingers until the mixture resembles pea-sized crumbs.
4. In a small bowl, whisk together the milk, brown sugar and honey. Add to the flour mixture and stir until the dough forms a ball.
5. Divide the dough into 2 equal balls.
6. On a lightly floured surface, roll out 1 ball to ⅛-inch (3 mm) thickness.
7. Cut into 2-inch (5 cm) squares or cut with a cookie cutter.
8. Prick the cracker tops with a fork and place them on ungreased baking sheets.
9. Repeat with the other ball of dough.
10. Bake for 12 to 15 minutes or until golden brown.
11. Remove from the oven. Remove the crackers from the baking sheet and cool on a rack.

These can be stored in a baking tin on the counter for 1 to 2 weeks or frozen for up to 3 months.

CHEESE & FLAX DIAMONDS

1½ cups (375 mL) shredded aged
  cheddar cheese

¾ cup (175 mL) soft margarine

1¼ cups (300 mL) unbleached
  all-purpose flour

¼ cup (50 mL) whole flaxseed

1 tsp (5 mL) dried mustard

¼ tsp (1 mL) onion or garlic powder

pinch cayenne pepper

YIELD: 48 diamonds

NUTRIENT VALUES PER
SERVING (1 DIAMOND)

Calories	57
Protein	1.5 g
Carbohydrates	3.0 g
Fibre	0.3 g
Fat	4.4 g
Saturated	1.3 g
Monounsaturated	1.5 g
Polyunsaturated	1.3 g
Cholesterol	4 mg
Folate	N/A
Potassium	22 mg
Sodium	61 mg

1. In a large bowl, using an electric mixer, beat together the cheese and margarine until light and almost smooth.

2. Stir in the flour, flaxseed, dried mustard, onion powder and cayenne pepper.

3. Divide the dough into 2 balls, cover and refrigerate for half an hour.

4. Preheat the oven to 375°F (190°C).

5. Roll out each ball on a lightly floured clean work surface to ⅛-inch (3 mm) thickness, about a 9- × 11-inch (23 × 28 cm) rectangle.

6. Cut into diamond shapes.

7. Place on ungreased baking sheets.

8. Bake for 10 to 12 minutes.

9. Remove from the oven and transfer to a rack to cool.

These can be stored in an airtight container for up to 3 days or frozen for up to 3 months.

FLAXSEED CRACKERS

1½ cups (375 mL) unbleached
all-purpose flour
¼ cup (50 mL) whole flaxseed
¼ cup (50 mL) ground flaxseed
½ tsp (2 mL) baking powder

½ tsp (2 mL) salt
4 tsp (20 mL) margarine or butter,
softened
½ cup (125 mL) skim milk

YIELD: 24 crackers

NUTRIENT VALUES PER
SERVING (1 CRACKER)

Calories	56
Protein	1.7 g
Carbohydrates	7.9 g
Fibre	0.9 g
Fat	1.9 g
Saturated	0.2 g
Monounsaturated	0.5 g
Polyunsaturated	1.1 g
Cholesterol	N/A
Folate	14 mcg
Potassium	66 mg
Sodium	59 mg

1. In the bowl of a stand mixer, combine the flour, whole and ground flaxseed, baking powder, salt and margarine. Using the paddle attachment, mix on low speed until the mixture resembles a coarse meal.
2. Add the milk and continue mixing to form a soft dough. You can also mix the dough by hand, if you prefer.
3. Wrap the dough in plastic wrap and refrigerate for 10 minutes.
4. Preheat the oven to 325°F (160°C).
5. Divide the dough into quarters. Turn out onto a lightly floured board. Roll each quarter out into a rectangle ¹⁄₁₆ inch (2 mm) thick. Cut into 2½-inch (6 cm) squares.
6. Transfer to an ungreased baking sheet.
7. Bake for 20 minutes or until crisp and golden.
8. Remove from the oven and transfer to a rack to cool.

These can be stored in an airtight container for up to 1 week or frozen for up to 3 months.

Adding just one or two ingredients can make for a tasty variation:
Onion   1 Tbsp (15 mL) powdered onion soup mix
Cheese   1 cup (250 mL) grated cheddar cheese
Italian   1 Tbsp (15 mL) dried oregano and 1 cup (250 mL) grated mozzarella cheese

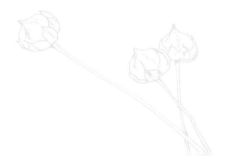

PEPPERY FLAX CRACKERS

3 cups (750 mL) whole wheat flour

⅔ cup (150 mL) ground flaxseed

⅓ cup (75 mL) whole flaxseed

1 Tbsp (15 mL) coarsely ground
black pepper

1 Tbsp (15 mL) steak spice

1 tsp (10 mL) salt

1½ cups (375 mL) warm water
(100 to 110°F/40 to 45°C)

coarse salt (optional)

YIELD: 8 large round crackers

NUTRIENT VALUES PER
SERVING (¼ CRACKER)

Calories	60
Protein	2.6 g
Carbohydrates	10.2 g
Fibre	2.7 g
Fat	2.0 g
Saturated	0.8 g
Monounsaturated	0.5 g
Polyunsaturated	0.6 g
Cholesterol	0 mg
Folate	5 mcg
Potassium	83 mg
Sodium	159 mg

INSTEAD OF WHOLE
WHEAT FLOUR, you can
use 2½ cups (625 mL) all-
purpose flour and 1 cup
(250 mL) bran.

INSTEAD OF THE PEPPER
AND STEAK SPICE, you can
use 4 tsp (20 mL) Montreal
Steak Spice.

1. Line 2 baking sheets with parchment paper.
2. In the bowl of a food processor, combine the flour, ground and whole flaxseed, pepper, steak spice and salt. Process for 10 seconds.
3. Add the water all at once and run the processor until the dough forms a ball (about 20 seconds).
4. Adjust the dough with water or flour, 1 Tbsp (15 mL) at a time, to make a smooth dough that is no longer sticky to the touch.
5. Process for an additional 60 seconds (to knead). Put the dough in a plastic bag or covered bowl and let it rest on the counter for half an hour.
6. Preheat the oven to 400°F (200°C).
7. Cut the dough into 8 pieces and roll each out into a 9-inch (23 cm) circle. Place the crackers on the prepared baking sheets.
8. Spray the crackers with water and sprinkle with coarse salt or additional spice if desired.
9. Bake for 10 to 18 minutes or until blistered, lightly browned and crisp. Check frequently as the crackers darken and crisp quite quickly near the end.
10. Remove from the oven and serve whole or broken.

These can be stored at room temperature in plastic wrap, bags or covered tins for up to 1 week. You may also cut the dough into triangles before baking, or deep-fry the triangles to make tortilla chip–style crackers.

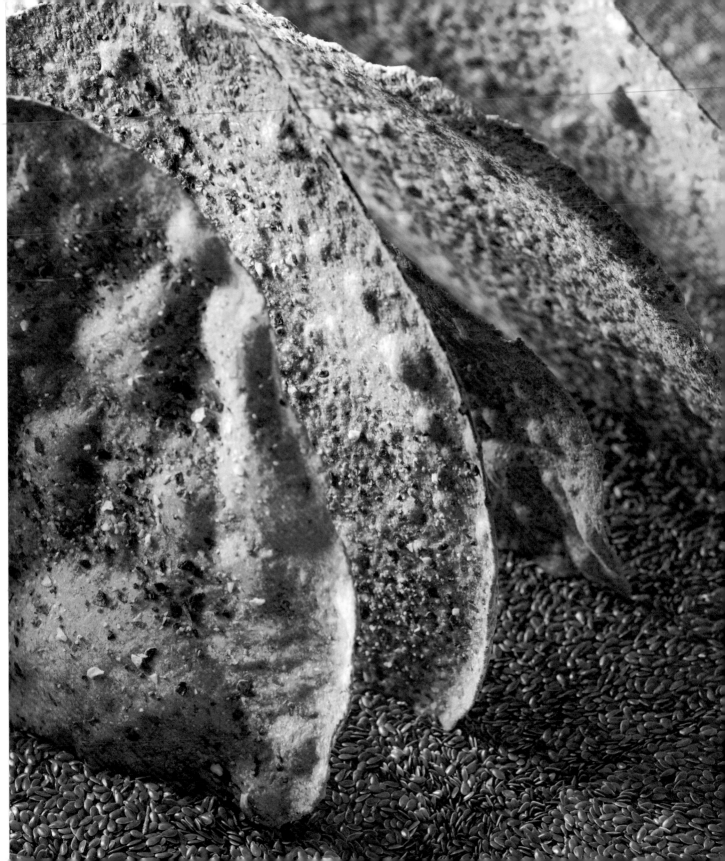

FLAX BRUSCHETTA-CROSTINI

1 multi-grain baguette, cut into
   ¾-inch (2 cm) slices

¼ tsp (1 mL) flaxseed oil per slice

1 cup (250 mL) diced onion

2 Tbsp (25 mL) flaxseed oil

2 Tbsp (25 mL) butter

2 cloves garlic, minced

½ tsp (2 mL) crushed dried basil

½ tsp (2 mL) crushed dried oregano

¼ tsp (1 mL) salt

pinch black pepper

5½ oz (156 mL) can tomato paste

⅓ cup (75 mL) whole toasted flaxseed

1 tsp (5 mL) shredded mozzarella
   cheese per slice

YIELD: 1½ cups (375 mL)
filling

NUTRIENT VALUES PER
SERVING (TWO ¾-INCH/
2 CM SLICES WITH
1 TBSP/15 ML OF FILL-
ING AND 1 TSP/5 ML OF
CHEESE PER SLICE)

Calories	363
Protein	14.7 g
Carbohydrates	49.5 g
Fibre	10.7 g
Fat	13.9 g
Saturated	2.1 g
Monounsaturated	1.5 g
Polyunsaturated	3.6 g
Cholesterol	7 mg
Folate	8 mcg
Potassium	197 mg
Sodium	619 mg

1. Preheat the oven to 375°F (190°C).
2. Place the sliced bread on a baking sheet. Drizzle ¼ tsp (1 mL) of flaxseed oil over each slice. Bake for 10 minutes, then remove from the oven.
3. Reduce the oven temperature to 275°F (140°C).
4. In a saucepan, combine the onion, flaxseed oil, butter, garlic, basil, oregano, salt and pepper. Cook over medium-low heat until bubbling. Reduce the heat, cover and simmer for 10 minutes or until the onion is just turning soft.
5. Stir in the tomato paste.
6. Remove from the heat and stir in the toasted flaxseed.
7. Place 1 Tbsp (15 mL) of filling on each toasted slice of bread and sprinkle with 1 tsp (5 mL) cheese.
8. Bake for 10 minutes or until the cheese has melted. Remove from the oven and serve immediately.

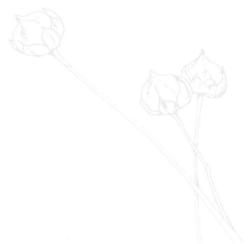

MINI CHEESEBALLS

1 cup (250 mL) grated medium
  cheddar cheese
4 oz (125 g) cream cheese, softened
2 Tbsp + 1 tsp (30 mL) Miracle Whip

1 tsp (5 mL) Worcestershire sauce
½ tsp (2 mL) Dijon mustard
whole flaxseed
pretzel sticks for garnish

YIELD: 10 to 12 cheeseballs

NUTRIENT VALUES PER
SERVING (2 BALLS)

Calories	240
Protein	9.0 g
Carbohydrates	5.2 g
Fibre	2.1 g
Fat	20.8 g
Saturated	10.4 g
Monounsaturated	4.9 g
Polyunsaturated	2.2 g
Cholesterol	51 mg
Folate	30 mcg
Potassium	106 mg
Sodium	290 mg

1. In a bowl, combine the cheddar cheese, cream cheese, Miracle Whip, Worcestershire sauce and Dijon mustard. Mix well.
2. Refrigerate for at least 1 hour or overnight.
3. Form the mixture into 1¼-inch (3 cm) balls.
4. Roll each ball in whole flaxseed to coat.
5. Put a pretzel in the middle of each ball.
6. Refrigerate for at least 2 hours or until ready to serve.

These can be stored in the refrigerator for up to 3 days.

CRACKED PEPPER & FLAX CHEESEBALLS

8 oz (250 g) light cream cheese

1 tsp (5 mL) cracked or coarsely
ground black pepper

1 tsp (5 mL) salt-free herb and spice
seasoning

2 Tbsp (25 mL) whole flaxseed

YIELD: 2 small cheeseballs
(about 1 cup/250 mL each)

NUTRIENT VALUES PER
SERVING (2 TSP/10 ML)

Calories	14
Protein	0.6 g
Carbohydrates	0.6 g
Fibre	0.1 g
Fat	1.0 g
Saturated	0.6 g
Monounsaturated	0 g
Polyunsaturated	0.1 g
Cholesterol	2 mg
Folate	2 mcg
Potassium	34 mg
Sodium	24 mg

1. In a medium bowl, mix together the cream cheese, pepper and seasoning with a fork until blended.
2. Divide into 2 balls.
3. In a small bowl, put 1 Tbsp (15 mL) flaxseed. Add 1 cheeseball, turning to coat all sides with seeds. Repeat with the other ball with the rest of the flaxseed.
4. Wrap each cheeseball with plastic wrap and refrigerate for 2 hours.

Serve with crackers and vegetables.

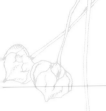

FLAX TOMATO CHEESEBALL

2 cups (500 mL) water

3 Tbsp (45 mL) sun-dried tomatoes

½ cup (125 mL) grated Parmesan
  cheese

½ cup (125 mL) cream cheese

½ cup (125 mL) butter

¼ cup (50 mL) ground toasted
  golden flaxseed

¼ cup (50 mL) crushed dried basil

1 Tbsp (15 mL) olive oil

½ tsp (2 mL) salt

YIELD: 1 medium cheeseball
(about 1½ cups/375 mL)

NUTRIENT VALUES PER
SERVING (2 TSP/10 ML)

Calories	48
Protein	1.1 g
Carbohydrates	0.7 g
Fibre	0.4 g
Fat	4.7 g
Saturated	2.7 g
Monounsaturated	1.5 g
Polyunsaturated	0.3 g
Cholesterol	12 mg
Folate	1 mcg
Potassium	33 mg
Sodium	97 mg

1. Bring the water to a boil, then add the sun-dried tomatoes. Boil for 3 minutes to rehydrate. Remove the tomatoes from the water. Cool them on a paper towel to absorb any excess water, then dice.
2. In a small food processor, combine the diced tomatoes, Parmesan cheese, cream cheese, butter, flaxseed, basil, oil and salt.
3. Process on the highest speed for 2 minutes or until the mixture has a smooth consistency.
4. Turn out the mixture onto a piece of plastic wrap and shape it into a ball.
5. Refrigerate for 2 hours or until set.
6. Remove from the refrigerator, unmold, unwrap and garnish as desired.

Serve with crackers and vegetables.

SALMON FLAX CHEESEBALL

Flax Fact: Just over one of every four farms in Saskatchewan include flax as part of their rotation.

8 oz (250 g) cream cheese, softened

⅔ cup (150 mL) butter, softened

½ cup (125 mL) shredded mozzarella cheese

⅓ cup (75 mL) ground toasted golden flaxseed

¼ cup (50 mL) smoked salmon

2 Tbsp (25 mL) finely chopped fresh cilantro

1 tsp (5 mL) brown sugar

½ tsp (2 mL) salt

pinch ground celery seed

¼ cup (50 mL) chopped raw pistachio nuts, plus extra for garnish (optional)

YIELD: 1 large cheeseball (about 2 cups)

NUTRIENT VALUES PER SERVING (2 TSP/10 ML)

Calories	49
Protein	1.0 g
Carbohydrates	0.7 g
Fibre	0.3 g
Fat	4.9 g
Saturated	2.8 g
Monounsaturated	1.5 g
Polyunsaturated	0.4 g
Cholesterol	14 mg
Folate	1 mcg
Potassium	22 mg
Sodium	71 mg

1. In a small food processor, place the cream cheese, butter, cheese, flaxseed, salmon, cilantro, brown sugar, salt and celery seed. Purée for 1 minute or until the mixture is smooth. Scrape down the sides of the bowl and process for another 30 seconds.
2. Stir in the pistachio nuts if using.
3. Turn out the mixture onto a piece of plastic wrap and shape it into a ball.
4. Refrigerate for 2 hours.
5. Remove from the refrigerator and remove the wrap.
6. Garnish with more pistachio nuts if desired.

Serve with assorted crackers.

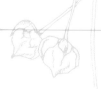

MUSHROOM BRUSCHETTA TOPPING

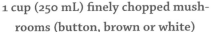

1 cup (250 mL) finely chopped mushrooms (button, brown or white)

¼ cup (50 mL) flaxseed oil

2 Tbsp (25 mL) balsamic vinegar

2 Tbsp (25 mL) finely chopped
   fresh basil

1 green onion, thinly sliced

1 clove garlic, minced

salt

black pepper

YIELD: 1 cup (250 mL)

NUTRIENT VALUES PER
SERVING (¼ CUP/50 ML)

Calories	113
Protein	0.7 g
Carbohydrates	2.4 g
Fibre	0.4 g
Fat	11.5 g
Saturated	1.1 g
Monounsaturated	2.0 g
Polyunsaturated	7.9 g
Cholesterol	0 mg
Folate	3 mcg
Potassium	89 mg
Sodium	241 mg

1. In a bowl, mix the mushrooms, flaxseed oil, vinegar, basil, onion and garlic.
2. Season with salt and pepper.
3. Let sit for 15 minutes to blend the flavours.
4. Spoon into a serving dish.

Double the recipe to serve with Onion & Olive Focaccia (page 62) or Ancient Grain Crackers (page 71).

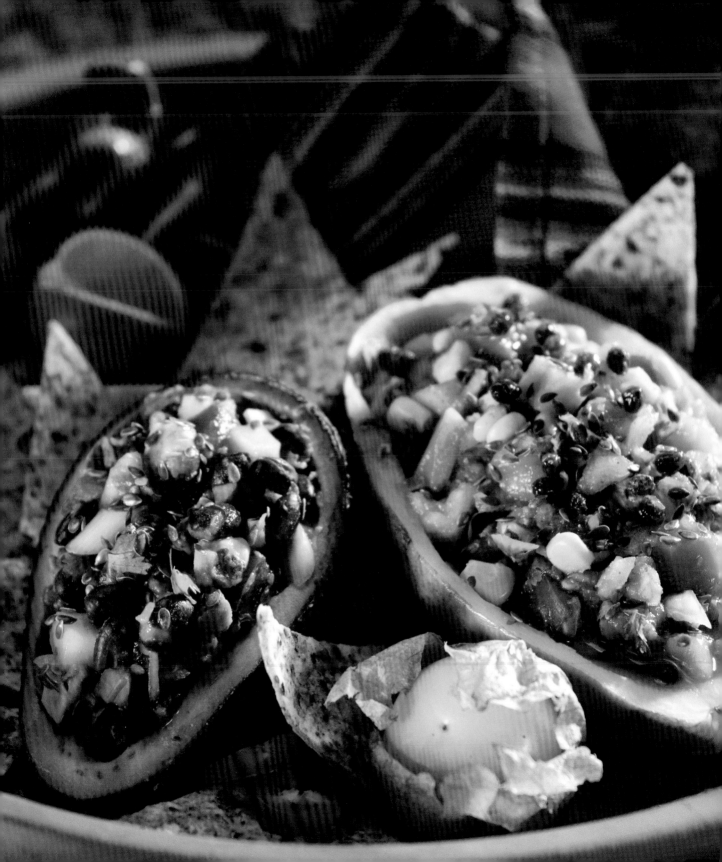

SUMMERTIME SALSA

YIELD: 4¾ cups (1.175 L)

NUTRIENT VALUES PER
SERVING (⅓ CUP/75 ML)

Calories	55
Protein	2.7 g
Carbohydrates	10.5 g
Fibre	3.6 g
Fat	1.7 g
Saturated	0.7 g
Monounsaturated	0.5 g
Polyunsaturated	0.5 g
Cholesterol	7 mg
Folate	208 mcg
Potassium	247 mg
Sodium	247 mg

19 oz (540 mL) can black beans, rinsed and drained
1 mango, peeled and chopped
1 cup (250 mL) seeded, diced Roma tomatoes
½ cup (125 mL) chopped red onion
⅓ cup (75 mL) sliced green onions
3 Tbsp (45 mL) fresh lime juice
2 Tbsp (25 mL) chopped fresh cilantro
2 Tbsp (25 mL) chopped fresh mint
1 tsp (5 mL) finely minced garlic
½ tsp (2 mL) salt
⅓ cup (75 mL) whole toasted flaxseed

1. In a bowl, combine the beans, mango, tomatoes, red and green onions, lime juice, cilantro, mint, garlic and salt. Mix well.
2. Cover and refrigerate for 2 hours.
3. Just before serving, stir in the flaxseed.

Serve with taco chips or use as a side dish or topping for a baked potato.

FIESTA SALSA

YIELD: 2 cups (500 mL)

NUTRIENT VALUES PER
SERVING (⅓ CUP/75 ML)

Calories	46
Protein	1.7 g
Carbohydrates	7.4 g
Fibre	2.4 g
Fat	2.2 g
Saturated	0.9 g
Monounsaturated	0.6 g
Polyunsaturated	0.6 g
Cholesterol	0 mg
Folate	12 mcg
Potassium	134 mg
Sodium	11 mg

1 cup (250 mL) diced papaya
½ cup (125 mL) frozen or fresh corn kernels
2 Tbsp (25 mL) finely diced sweet onion
1 Roma tomato, diced
1 jalapeño pepper, minced
1 clove garlic, minced
2 Tbsp (25 mL) fresh lime juice
1 tsp (5 mL) grated lime zest
3 Tbsp (45 mL) ground flaxseed
2 Tbsp (25 mL) chopped fresh cilantro
2 tsp (10 mL) whole flaxseed

1. In a medium bowl, toss together the papaya, corn, onion, tomato, jalapeño, garlic, lime juice and zest. Cover and refrigerate for 2 hours.
2. Just before serving, stir in the ground flaxseed, cilantro and whole flaxseed.

Serve with chips or crackers or use as a side dish or topping for a baked potato.

CALIFORNIA SUSHI ROLLS

Flax Fact: In the vegetable garden, flax is a good companion crop for carrots and potatoes, improving both growth and flavour.

2 cups (500 mL) medium-grain sushi rice

3 cups (750 mL) water

1 tsp (5 mL) salt

¼ cup (50 mL) whole flaxseed

¼ cup (50 mL) seasoned rice vinegar

2 tsp (10 mL) cooking sherry (optional)

1 ripe avocado, peeled, cut into 8 wedges

one 7-inch (18 cm) length of English cucumber, peeled, cut in half lengthwise

six 5-inch (12 cm) imitation crab sticks

4 sheets nori (seaweed)

bamboo sushi mat

YIELD: 32 sushi rolls

NUTRIENT VALUES PER SERVING (4 ROLLS)

Calories	349
Protein	13.8 g
Carbohydrates	58.7 g
Fibre	3.3 g
Fat	6.6 g
Saturated	1.6 g
Monounsaturated	3.1 g
Polyunsaturated	1.4 g
Cholesterol	31 mg
Folate	113 mcg
Potassium	420 mg
Sodium	477 mg

BAMBOO SUSHI MATS can be purchased in the ethnic section of large supermarkets.

1. Rinse the rice well in cold water and drain.
2. In a 6-cup (1.5 L) saucepan, combine the rice, water and salt. Cover and bring to a boil over high heat.
3. Reduce to low heat and simmer for 20 to 25 minutes, or until the water is absorbed.
4. Gently fold in the flaxseed, seasoned rice vinegar and cooking sherry (if using). Cool to room temperature.
5. Take one half of the cucumber and cut it lengthwise into 4 wedges. Reserve the other half for another use.
6. Lay the bamboo mat on a clean work surface with the slats parallel to the edge. Place 1 nori sheet on the top short end, shiny side down.
7. Spread 1¼ cups (300 mL) of the rice to a ¼-inch (6 mm) thickness on the nori, leaving a ½-inch (1 cm) edge at the top.
8. Lay 2 pieces of avocado end to end, 1 cucumber spear and 1½ crab sticks end to end on the lower third of the rice. Using your thumb, push the bamboo mat edge nearest you up and over the filling, holding the row of ingredients in place with your fingertips.

Continued on page 94 . . .

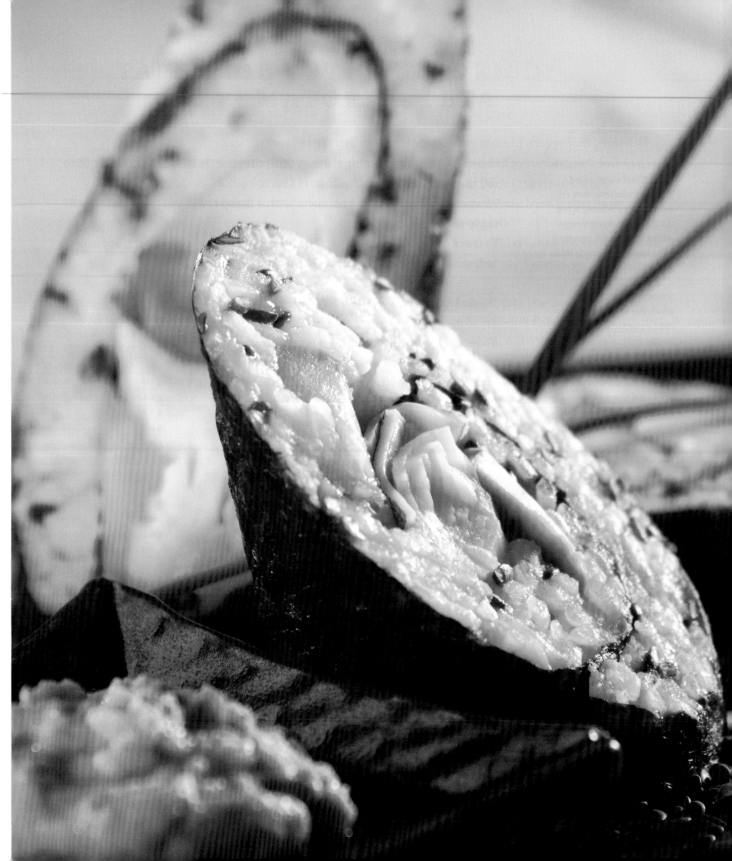

ASIAN SALAD ROLLS

12 sheets round 9-inch (23 cm)
diameter rice paper

3½ oz (100 g) packet dried rice
vermicelli noodles

¾ cup (175 mL) ground flaxseed,
about 1 Tbsp (15 mL) per roll

¾ cup (175 mL) whole flaxseed,
about 1 Tbsp (15 mL) per roll

12 butter lettuce or leaf lettuce
leaves, shredded

12 chives or green onions, cut
into thirds

12 sprigs fresh cilantro

deli sprouts

soy ginger sauce

YIELD: 12 rolls

NUTRIENT VALUES PER
SERVING (1 ROLL)

Calories	215
Protein	8.0 g
Carbohydrates	33.1 g
Fibre	6.6 g
Fat	8.6 g
Saturated	3.5 g
Monounsaturated	2.3 g
Polyunsaturated	2.6 g
Cholesterol	3 mg
Folate	47 mcg
Potassium	249 mg
Sodium	211 mg

1. Soften the rice paper by soaking the sheets in a pan of warm water until moistened. Remove, pat dry and lay flat on a clean, dry cloth. Leave for 15 seconds or until pliable. Use immediately or stack between waxed paper until needed.

2. Soak the dried noodles in hot water for 10 minutes, then place them in boiling water for 2 to 4 minutes. Drain. Rinse under cold water. Pat dry.

3. Lay 1 sheet of softened rice paper at a time on a clean, damp cloth.

4. Layer the vermicelli noodles, ground and whole flaxseed, lettuce, chives, a sprig of cilantro, deli sprouts and soy ginger sauce to taste on the rice paper. Roll and fold in the ends. Set aside and cover with a clean, moistened cloth or towel. Top with more ginger sauce. Continue until all the rice paper is used. Serve.

Shrimp, crab-flavoured pollock or prosciutto ham can be added on the rice paper before the veggies and flaxseed.

MAYAN MIX
CHILI-CHEESE MUNCHIES

2 cups (500 mL) whole grain wheat squares cereal

1½ cups (375 mL) whole grain flaked cereal (see sidebar)

1½ cups (375 mL) puffed kamut (see sidebar)

1½ cups (375 mL) toasted oat cereal

1 cup (250 mL) unsalted mixed nuts

½ cup (125 mL) raw, shelled pumpkin seeds

⅓ cup (75 mL) flaxseed oil

¼ cup (50 mL) cheddar cheese powder

4 tsp (20 mL) chili or taco seasoning

1 Tbsp (15 mL) Worcestershire sauce

YIELD: 8 cups (2 L)

NUTRIENT VALUES PER
SERVING (½ CUP/125 ML)

Calories	208
Protein	5.6 g
Carbohydrates	16.3 g
Fibre	2.4 g
Fat	14.4 g
Saturated	2.2 g
Monounsaturated	5.2 g
Polyunsaturated	5.6 g
Cholesterol	1 mg
Folate	19 mcg
Potassium	185 mg
Sodium	258 mg

KAMUT is a high-protein wheat, found as a whole grain, flour or puffed cereal.

WHOLE GRAIN FLAKED CEREAL can be bought wherever organic foods are sold.

1. In a large plastic container with a tight-fitting lid, combine the wheat squares, flaked cereal, kamut, oat cereal, nuts and pumpkin seeds.

2. In a jar with a tight-fitting lid, combine the flaxseed oil, cheese powder, seasoning and Worcestershire sauce. Shake well, then drizzle over the cereal mixture.

3. Seal the container with its lid. Shake well to coat the mixture.

4. Let set for 2 hours before serving.

Store in a plastic container for up to 1 week.

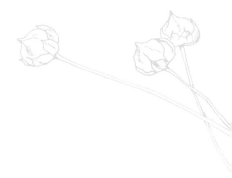

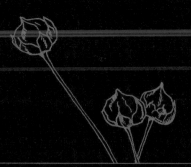

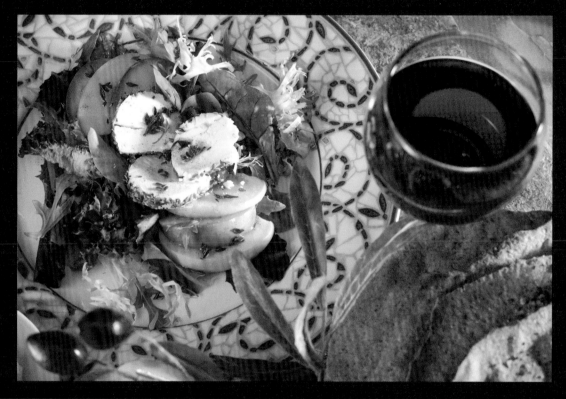

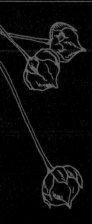

Pictured: *Flax-Coated Goat Cheese & Apple Salad* (page 118)

Soups, Salads & More

Ah . . . soup. It's the ultimate in wholesome quality, particularly when flax is included in the recipe! For hearty soups like the Peasant Soup with Flax Farfel, or the Lentil Soup with Orzo, all you need for a complete meal is bread, a salad or fresh fruit. The soup shooters are an imaginative teaser for the main dish to follow, but be prepared for requests to refill that glass a second or third time!

Salads can be colourful and nutritious, and an inspiring way to achieve healthy eating no matter what your schedule, lifestyle and dietary needs are like. This collection of salad recipes, from the always popular Spinach Strawberry to the basic Broccoli to the more formal Flax-Coated Goat Cheese and Apple Salad, is presented for your enjoyment. Flaxseed and/or flaxseed oil help bring out the goodness, taste and texture of these exciting salads.

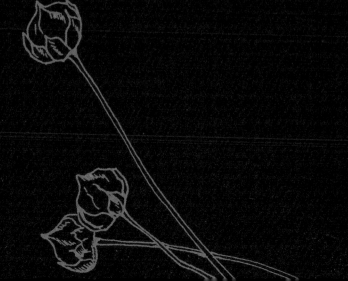

CURRIED POTATO SOUP

3 strips bacon

1 cup (250 mL) diced onion

3 cups (750 mL) diced potato

1 tsp (5 mL) curry powder

¼ cup (50 mL) low-sodium chicken
   soup base or 3 bouillon cubes

2 cups (500 mL) boiling water

½ cup (125 mL) whole flaxseed

½ cup (125 mL) coconut milk

½ cup (125 mL) frozen peas

YIELD: 6 cups (1.5 L)

NUTRIENT VALUES PER
SERVING (1 CUP/250 ML)

Calories	203
Protein	6.9 g
Carbohydrates	22.3 g
Fibre	5.8 g
Fat	10.6 g
Saturated	4.8 g
Monounsaturated	1.9 g
Polyunsaturated	3.3 g
Cholesterol	3 mg
Folate	62 mcg
Potassium	606 mg
Sodium	788 mg

1. In a small non-stick skillet over medium heat, fry the bacon until crisp.

2. Place the bacon on a sheet of paper towel, reserving 2 Tbsp (25 mL) drippings. Blot well.

3. In a 10-cup (2.5 L) saucepan, sauté the onion in the reserved bacon drippings for 5 minutes.

4. Add the diced potato and curry powder. Cook, stirring, for 1 minute.

5. Dissolve the chicken base in the boiling water and stir. Add to the potato mixture, cover and simmer over medium-low heat for 20 minutes, or until the potatoes are tender.

6. In the same small non-stick skillet, toast the flaxseed over medium heat, covered, until the seeds begin to pop. Remove from the heat.

7. Add the coconut milk and peas to the soup. Cover and cook over medium heat until hot and steaming.

8. Dice the bacon and add it to the soup.

9. Sprinkle with the toasted flaxseed and serve.

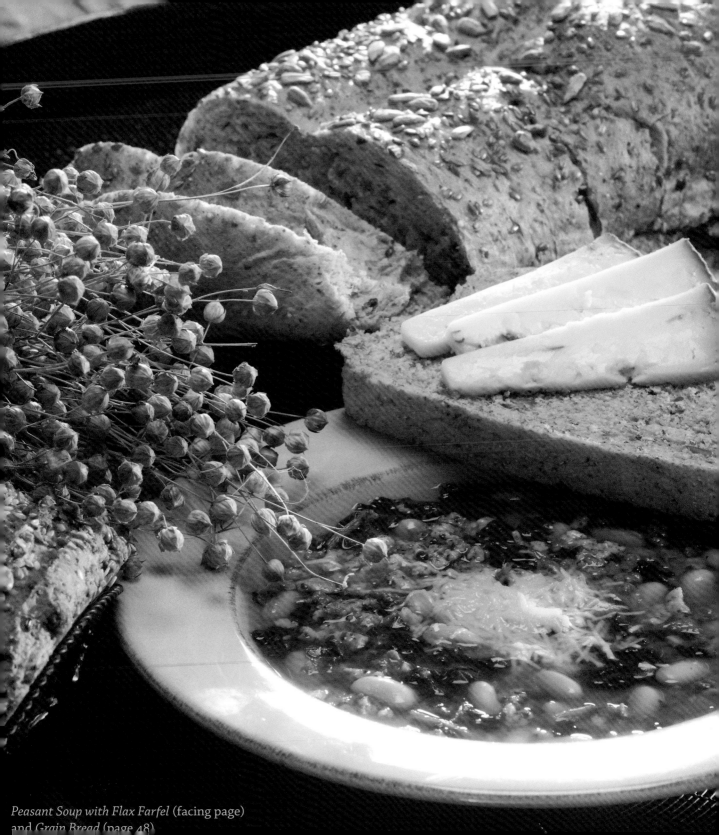

Peasant Soup with Flax Farfel (facing page)
and *Grain Bread* (page 48)

PEASANT SOUP WITH FLAX FARFEL

1 lb (500 g) lean ground beef or any
    fresh ground meat
¼ cup (50 mL) finely chopped onion
2 cloves garlic, minced
1 tsp (5 mL) crushed dried basil
½ tsp (2 mL) crushed dried oregano
8 cups (2 L) chicken stock
1 cup (250 mL) dried farfel
    or 1¼ cups (300 mL) fresh farfel
    (see recipe below)

19 oz (540 mL) can white kidney beans,
    rinsed and drained
8 oz (250 g) package frozen chopped
    spinach, thawed, squeezed dry
2 Tbsp (25 mL) ketchup
freshly grated Parmesan cheese

YIELD: 12 cups (3 L)

NUTRIENT VALUES PER
SERVING (1 CUP/250 ML)

Calories	187
Protein	15.0 g
Carbohydrates	18.4 g
Fibre	3.9 g
Fat	6.5 g
Saturated	2.5 g
Monounsaturated	2.5 g
Polyunsaturated	0.9 g
Cholesterol	51 mg
Folate	77 mcg
Potassium	397 mg
Sodium	577 mg

1. Sauté the meat in a large saucepan over medium heat until almost all the pink is gone, about 7 minutes.
2. Drain off any fat.
3. Add the onion, garlic, basil and oregano. Stir and cook for 2 minutes.
4. Add the chicken stock. Bring to a boil over medium-high heat. Reduce the heat and simmer for 10 minutes.
5. Stir in the dried or fresh farfel and cook until done, about 15 minutes for dried, 7 minutes for fresh.
6. Add the beans, spinach and ketchup. Bring to a simmer and cook for 5 minutes, stirring occasionally.
7. Serve with freshly grated Parmesan cheese.

Flax farfel

1 cup (250 mL) unbleached
    all-purpose flour
⅓ cup (75 mL) ground flaxseed

½ tsp (2 mL) salt
2 large eggs

YIELD: 1¼ cups (300 mL)
farfel

1. In a bowl, combine the flour, flaxseed and salt. Mix well. Turn the mixture out onto a clean work surface.
2. Make a well in the centre and break the eggs into the well.

Continued on the next page . . .

AUTUMN SQUASH SOUP
SHOOTER WITH SHERRY

6 Tbsp (100 mL) ground flaxseed

2 Tbsp (25 mL) canola oil

1 large onion, chopped

3½ lb (1.75 kg) frozen or fresh
   cooked cubed butternut squash

3 cups (750 mL) chicken stock,
   apple juice or water

1 cup (250 mL) buttermilk (see
   page 18)

½ tsp (2 mL) sea salt

¼ tsp (1 mL) ground white pepper

¼ cup (50 mL) dry sherry (optional)

YIELD: 20 shooters or
8 bowls

NUTRIENT VALUES PER
SERVING (1 SHOOTER)

Calories	69
Protein	1.8 g
Carbohydrates	11.2 g
Fibre	3.1 g
Fat	2.5 g
Saturated	0.3 g
Monounsaturated	N/A
Polyunsaturated	N/A
Cholesterol	1 mg
Folate	N/A
Potassium	N/A
Sodium	65 mg

1. Place the flaxseed in an ungreased heavy skillet. Cook, stirring, for 2 to 3 minutes on medium heat.

2. Add the oil and onion. Sauté until the onion is soft.

3. Add the squash and stock.

4. Cover and simmer for 40 minutes.

5. Remove from the heat and use a handheld blender to process the soup until smooth.

6. Whisk in the buttermilk, salt and pepper. Add the sherry if using.

7. Season to taste.

8. Reheat gently before serving. Do not boil.

9. Pour into individual shooter glasses (or bowls).

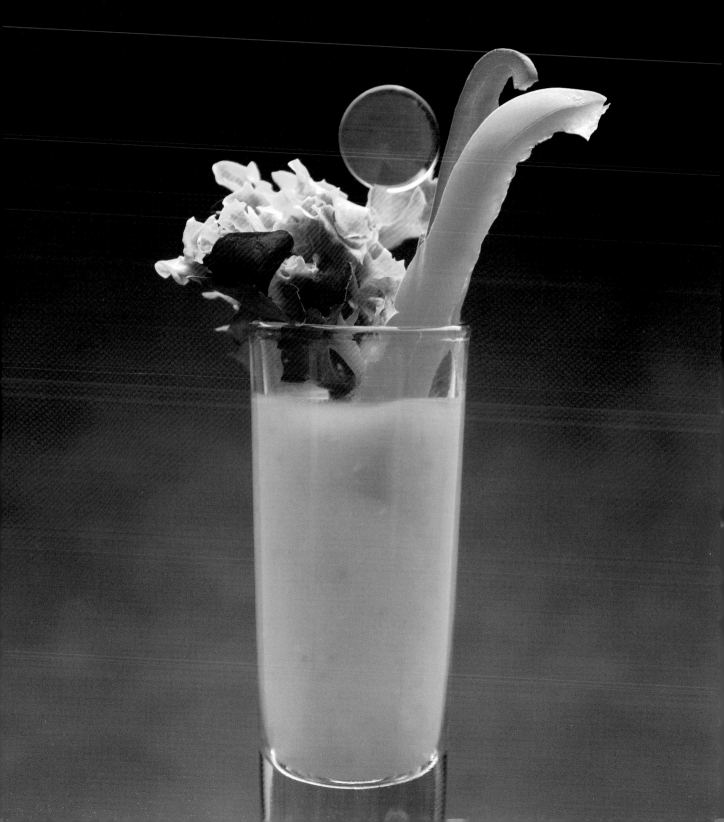

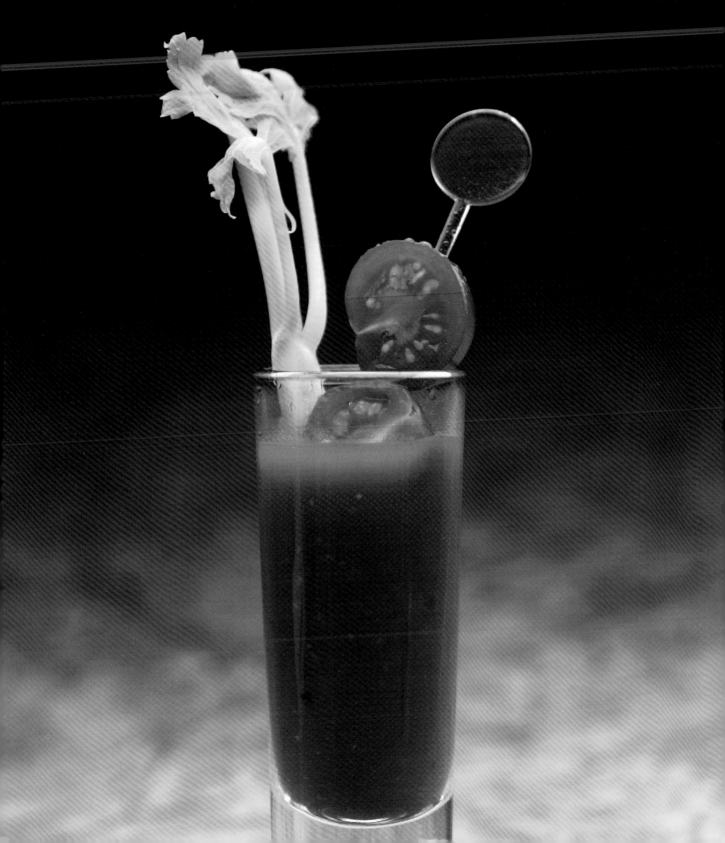

BLOODY MARY TOMATO SOUP SHOOTER

6 Tbsp (100 mL) ground flaxseed

2 Tbsp (25 mL) canola oil

1 large onion, chopped

4 stalks celery, finely chopped

1 Tbsp (15 mL) minced garlic

4 cups (1 L) tomato juice

2 cups (500 mL) canned diced
   tomatoes

2 cups (500 mL) water

½ cup (125 mL) chopped fresh parsley

1 tsp (5 mL) crushed red chili flakes

1 tsp (5 mL) sea salt

½ tsp (2 mL) black pepper

¼ cup (50 mL) vodka (optional)

dash Tabasco sauce (optional)

dash Worcestershire sauce (optional)

celery, halved cherry tomatoes and
   lemon slices for garnish (optional)

YIELD: 20 shooters or
8 bowls

NUTRIENT VALUES PER
SERVING (1 SHOOTER)

Calories	45
Protein	1.3 g
Carbohydrates	5.4 g
Fibre	1.7 g
Fat	2.4 g
Saturated	0.2 g
Monounsaturated	N/A
Polyunsaturated	N/A
Cholesterol	0 mg
Folate	N/A
Potassium	N/A
Sodium	165 mg

1. Place the flaxseed in an ungreased heavy skillet. Cook, stirring, for 2 to 3 minutes on medium heat.
2. Add the oil, onion, celery and garlic. Sauté until soft.
3. Add the tomato juice, tomatoes, water, parsley, chili flakes, salt and pepper. Bring to a boil.
4. Simmer gently for 20 minutes.
5. Remove from the heat and use a handheld blender to process until smooth.
6. Add the vodka, Tabasco and Worcestershire sauce if using.
7. Season to taste.
8. Reheat gently before serving. Do not boil.
9. Pour into individual shooter glasses (or bowls). Garnish with celery, cherry tomatoes and/or lemon slices if desired.

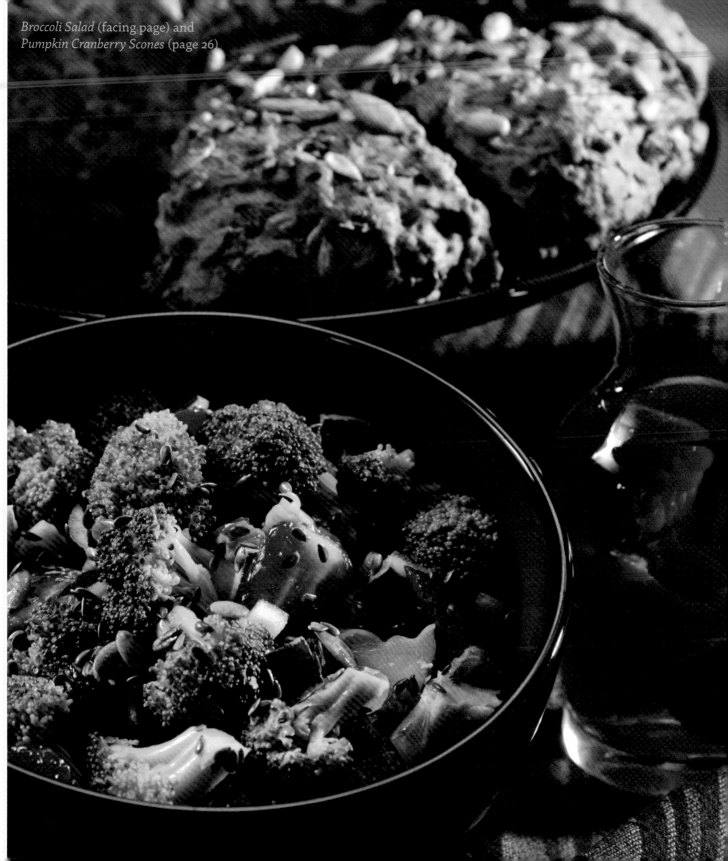

Broccoli Salad (facing page) and
Pumpkin Cranberry Scones (page 26)

BROCCOLI SALAD

Salad

6 cups (1.5 L) chopped broccoli

¾ cup (175 mL) cran-raisins or raisins

½ cup (125 mL) shelled, roasted pumpkin seeds

¼ cup (50 mL) finely chopped red onion

2 Tbsp (25 mL) whole flaxseed

Dressing

¾ cup (175 mL) light mayonnaise

2 Tbsp (25 mL) raspberry vinegar

2 Tbsp (25 mL) granulated sugar

YIELD: 6 servings

NUTRIENT VALUES PER SERVING (1 CUP/250 ML)

Calories	319
Protein	10.7 g
Carbohydrates	29.5 g
Fibre	4.3 g
Fat	20.1 g
Saturated	3.8 g
Monounsaturated	4.2 g
Polyunsaturated	7.7 g
Cholesterol	0 mg
Folate	92 mcg
Potassium	681 mg
Sodium	251 mg

INSTEAD OF THE PUMPKIN SEEDS, use sunflower seeds, chopped walnuts or nuts of your choice.

1. For the salad, in a large bowl, place the broccoli, cran-raisins, pumpkin seeds, onion and flaxseed.
2. For the dressing, in another bowl, combine the mayonnaise, vinegar and sugar. Mix well.
3. Pour the dressing over the salad and toss well.
4. Refrigerate before serving.

CURRIED RICE & GRAPE SALAD

1½ cups (375 mL) cooked brown
 rice, cooled
⅓ cup (75 mL) low-fat plain yogurt
2 Tbsp (25 mL) flaxseed oil
1 tsp (5 mL) curry powder
1 tsp (5 mL) granulated sugar
½ tsp (2 mL) salt

¼ tsp (1 mL) crushed dried mint or
 ground cinnamon
1½ cups (375 mL) halved seedless
 red or green grapes
2 Tbsp (25 mL) whole toasted
 flaxseed

YIELD: 6 servings

NUTRIENT VALUES PER
SERVING (½ CUP/125 ML)

Calories	140
Protein	2.8 g
Carbohydrates	18.6 g
Fibre	2.3 g
Fat	6.4 g
Saturated	0.7 g
Monounsaturated	1.2 g
Polyunsaturated	4.2 g
Cholesterol	N/A
Folate	16 mcg
Potassium	148 mg
Sodium	207 mg

1. In a medium bowl, combine the rice, yogurt, flaxseed oil, curry powder, sugar, salt and mint. Mix well.
2. Toss in the grapes.
3. Cover and refrigerate for 24 hours.
4. Mix in the toasted flaxseed just before serving.

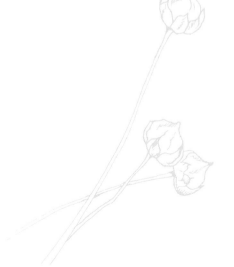

MARINATED GREEK SALAD

YIELD: 6 servings

NUTRIENT VALUES PER
SERVING (1 CUP/250 ML)

Calories	299
Protein	5.7 g
Carbohydrates	36.0 g
Fibre	6.7 g
Fat	24.6 g
Saturated	3.5 g
Monounsaturated	4.1 g
Polyunsaturated	8.3 g
Cholesterol	5 mg
Folate	78 mcg
Potassium	620 mg
Sodium	508 mg

⅔ cup (150 mL) bottled Greek with
   Feta and Oregano dressing
¼ cup (50 mL) flaxseed oil
6 cups (1.5 L) assorted vegetables
   (cauliflower, broccoli, pitted olives,
   grape tomatoes, cucumber, carrots)

¼ cup (50 mL) crumbled feta cheese
2 Tbsp (25 mL) whole toasted flaxseed
   per serving

1. In a bowl, combine the Greek dressing and flaxseed oil. Whisk together until well blended.
2. In another bowl, combine the vegetables. Pour the dressing over the vegetables and toss to coat.
3. Cover and refrigerate for 6 to 12 hours, tossing occasionally.
4. Just before serving, add the feta cheese and toss again.
5. Divide the salad into 6 dishes.
6. Sprinkle each serving with 2 Tbsp (25 mL) of toasted flaxseed.

MARINATED ITALIAN SALAD

YIELD: 6 servings

NUTRIENT VALUES PER
SERVING (1 CUP/250 ML)

Calories	285
Protein	5.0 g
Carbohydrates	16.2 g
Fibre	6.9 g
Fat	23.6 g
Saturated	2.4 g
Monounsaturated	3.8 g
Polyunsaturated	8.3 g
Cholesterol	0 mg
Folate	77 mcg
Potassium	625 mg
Sodium	606 mg

⅔ cup (150 mL) bottled Zesty
   Italian dressing
¼ cup (50 mL) flaxseed oil
6 cups (1.5 L) assorted vegetables
   (cauliflower, broccoli, pitted olives,
   grape tomatoes, cucumber, carrots)

1 Tbsp (15 mL) whole toasted
   flaxseed per serving

1. In a bowl, combine the Italian dressing and flaxseed oil. Whisk until well blended.
2. In another bowl, combine the vegetables. Pour the dressing over the vegetables and toss to coat.
3. Cover and refrigerate for 6 to 12 hours, tossing occasionally.
4. Divide the salad into 3 bowls.
5. Sprinkle each serving with 1 Tbsp (15 mL) of toasted flaxseed.

FLAX-COATED GOAT CHEESE & APPLE SALAD

Flax Fact: A unique feature of flaxseed is the high ratio of alpha-linolenic acid (an omega-3 fatty acid) to linoleic (an omega-6 fatty acid). Essential fatty acids are beneficial for cardiovascular health, inflammatory disorders, immunity and certain cancers.

Apple garnish

1 cup (250 mL) water

2 Tbsp (25 mL) fresh lemon juice

1 Tbsp (15 mL) granulated sugar

1 red apple, cored, sliced into 12 wedges

1 green apple, cored, sliced into 12 wedges

Dressing

¼ cup (50 mL) poaching liquid from apples

2 Tbsp (25 mL) pure maple syrup

1 Tbsp (15 mL) apple cider vinegar

1 Tbsp (15 mL) flaxseed oil

¼ tsp (1 mL) crushed dried thyme

pinch ground cinnamon

Salad

4 cups (1 L) packed baby greens (142 g bag)

5 oz (150 g) goat cheese roll

2 Tbsp (25 mL) whole flaxseed

YIELD: 4 servings

NUTRIENT VALUES PER SERVING (½ CUP/125 ML)

Calories	260
Protein	9.6 g
Carbohydrates	23.5 g
Fibre	4.5 g
Fat	16.0 g
Saturated	8.4 g
Monounsaturated	3.5 g
Polyunsaturated	3.3 g
Cholesterol	28 mg
Folate	69 mcg
Potassium	381 mg
Sodium	201 mg

1. In a large saucepan, bring the water, lemon juice and sugar to a boil.
2. Add the apple slices and gently poach them until they're tender-crisp, about 4 minutes.
3. Carefully lift out the apple slices with a slotted spoon. Set aside to cool. Reserve the poaching liquid.
4. In a small bowl, whisk together the poaching liquid, maple syrup, vinegar, flaxseed oil, thyme and cinnamon.
5. Divide the salad greens among 4 serving plates.
6. Roll the goat cheese in the flaxseed to coat it evenly. Cut it into 12 slices.
7. Place 3 slices of cheese on top of each salad portion.
8. Arrange 3 slices each of red and green apple on each salad portion.
9. Drizzle 2 Tbsp (25 mL) of salad dressing over each plate.

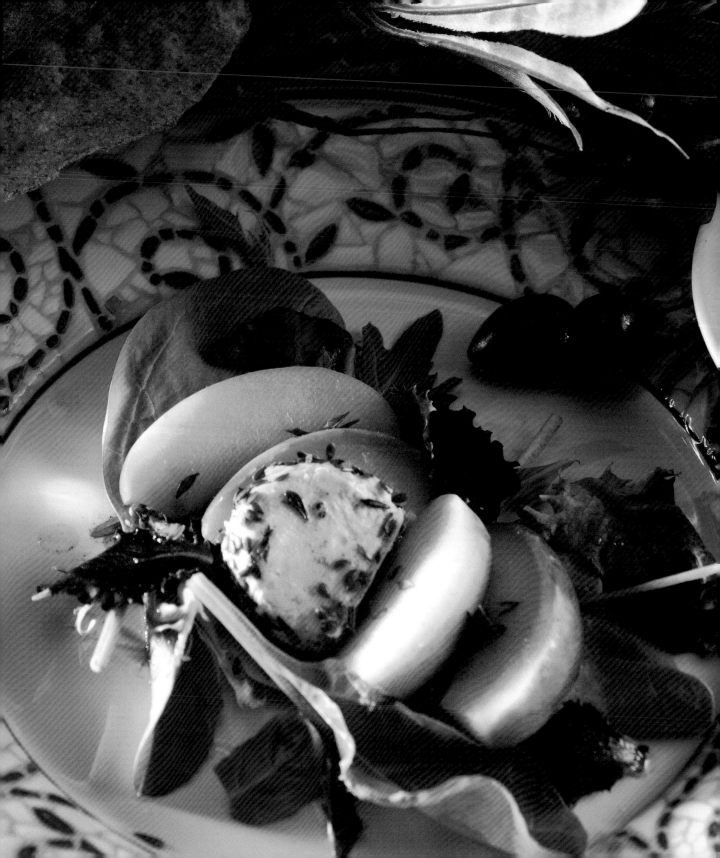

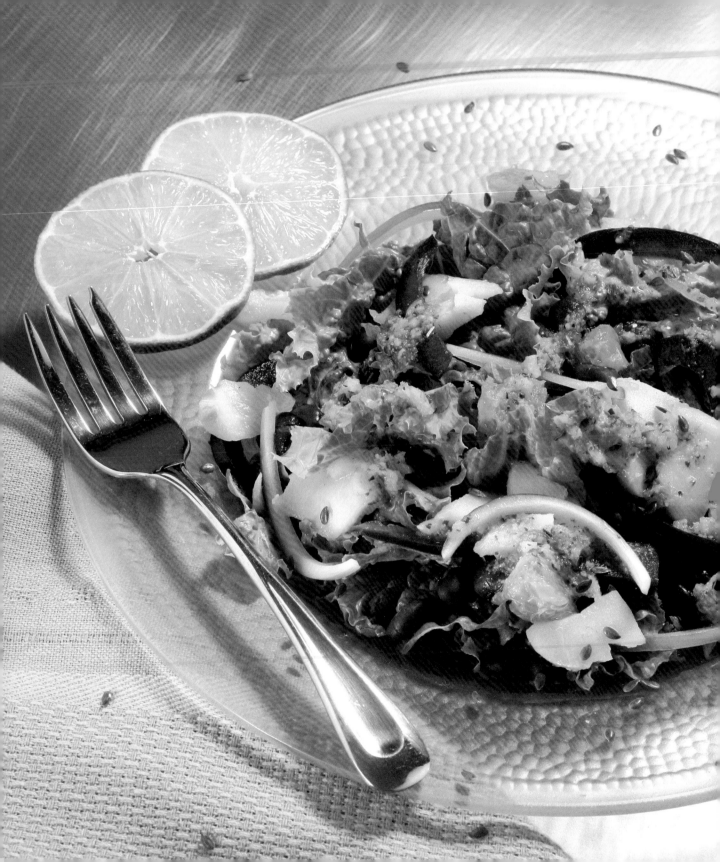

RED SNAPPER & BEAN SALAD WITH CUBAN MOJITO SAUCE

Flax Fact: "Flax" comes from an Indo-European word meaning "to plait." It was first used as a material rather than a foodstuff. Flax's given name, *Linum usitatissimum*, means "most used and most useful."

Mojito sauce

3 Tbsp (45 mL) fresh orange juice (about 1 orange)

1 Tbsp (15 mL) fresh lime juice (about ½ lime)

2 tsp (10 mL) grated lime zest (about ½ lime)

¼ cup (50 mL) flaxseed oil

2 tsp (10 mL) whole flaxseed

1 tsp (5 mL) sherry vinegar or red wine vinegar

2 cloves garlic, crushed

2 tsp (10 mL) freshly grated ginger

1 tsp (5 mL) crushed dried oregano

1 tsp (5 mL) granulated sugar

½ tsp (2 mL) ground cumin

½ tsp (2 mL) salt

Salad

2 oranges

1 lb (500 g) red snapper fillets

1 cup (250 mL) water

salt

black pepper

19 oz (540 mL) can black beans or black-eyed peas, rinsed and drained

3 cups (750 mL) torn spinach or lettuce

½ cup (125 mL) slivered red bell pepper

¼ cup (50 mL) slivered red onion

YIELD: 8 servings

NUTRIENT VALUES PER SERVING (1 CUP/250 ML)

Calories	199
Protein	19.4 g
Carbohydrates	18.7 g
Fibre	5.0 g
Fat	6.6 g
Saturated	0.9 g
Monounsaturated	1.2 g
Polyunsaturated	4.0 g
Cholesterol	27 mg
Folate	62 mcg
Potassium	753 mg
Sodium	507 mg

Based on recipe made with spinach and red wine vinegar

1. For the sauce, in a jar with a tight-fitting lid, combine the orange juice, lime juice, lime zest, flaxseed oil, whole flaxseed, vinegar, garlic, ginger, oregano, sugar, cumin and salt. Shake well.

2. For the salad, in a skillet with a lid, slice 1 orange into ¼-inch (6 mm) slices. Lay the orange slices in the bottom of the pan, then lay the snapper fillets overtop. Pour the water overtop, then season lightly with salt and pepper.

3. Bring to a boil, cover and reduce the heat to a simmer. Cook until the fish is opaque all the way through, about 10 minutes.

4. Carefully lift the fish out of the skillet. Let it cool on several layers of paper towel.

5. In a large salad bowl, combine the beans, spinach, bell pepper and onion.

6. Peel the remaining orange and separate it into segments. Cut each segment crosswise into 4 pieces. Add them to the salad.

7. Drizzle the mojito sauce over the salad and gently toss to coat.

8. Break the snapper into bite-sized pieces. Gently toss them into the salad.

RUSSIAN SALAD DRESSING

1 cup (250 mL) canned diced
   tomatoes
¼ cup (50 mL) red wine vinegar
2 Tbsp (25 mL) flaxseed oil
2 Tbsp (25 mL) brown sugar
1 tsp (5 mL) Worcestershire sauce

1 tsp (5 mL) seasoned salt
1 tsp (5 mL) paprika
1 tsp (5 mL) prepared horseradish
2 cloves garlic, minced
1 green onion, chopped

YIELD: 1½ cups (375 mL)

NUTRIENT VALUES PER
SERVING (2 TBSP/25 ML)

Calories	28
Protein	0.2 g
Carbohydrates	3.0 g
Fibre	0.3 g
Fat	1.8 g
Saturated	0.2 g
Monounsaturated	0.3 g
Polyunsaturated	1.3 g
Cholesterol	0 mg
Folate	1 mcg
Potassium	18 mg
Sodium	88 mg

1. Place the tomatoes, vinegar, flaxseed oil, brown sugar, Worcestershire sauce, salt, paprika, horseradish, garlic and green onion in a blender.
2. Blend until smooth, about 45 seconds.
3. Refrigerate the dressing in a sealed container for up to 1 week.

This dressing works well with any green salad and is also delicious on marinated vegetable salads.

SMOKED CHIPOTLE PEPPER TOPPING

YIELD: 3 Tbsp (45 mL)

NUTRIENT VALUES PER
SERVING (2 TSP/10 ML)

Calories	68
Protein	0.8 g
Carbohydrates	0.3 g
Fibre	0.1 g
Fat	7.3 g
Saturated	1.0 g
Monounsaturated	1.3 g
Polyunsaturated	4.7 g
Cholesterol	1 mg
Folate	2 mcg
Potassium	8 mg
Sodium	30 mg

Based on recipe made
without salt

2 Tbsp (25 mL) flaxseed oil
1 Tbsp (15 mL) grated Parmesan
  cheese
1 tsp (5 mL) finely chopped chives

½ tsp (2 mL) crushed dried
  chipotle pepper or bacon bits
pinch garlic powder
salt

1. In a small bowl, combine the flaxseed oil, Parmesan cheese, chives, chipotle pepper, garlic powder and salt to taste.
2. Let stand for at least 1 hour to allow the flavours to blend. Cover the bowl tightly and refrigerate for up to 1 week.

This topping is great drizzled on baked or boiled baby potatoes, steamed vegetables, pasta, bread, etc. Pictured on page 131.

MAPLE-PECAN TOPPING

YIELD: ¼ cup (50 mL)

NUTRIENT VALUES PER
SERVING (1 TBSP/15 ML)

Calories	114
Protein	0.2 g
Carbohydrates	4.7 g
Fibre	0.2 g
Fat	10.8 g
Saturated	1.0 g
Monounsaturated	2.6 g
Polyunsaturated	6.8 g
Cholesterol	0 mg
Folate	1 mcg
Potassium	23 mg
Sodium	1 mg

2 Tbsp (25 mL) flaxseed oil
1 Tbsp (15 mL) pure maple syrup

1 Tbsp (15 mL) finely chopped pecans
dash ground cinnamon

In a small bowl, combine the flaxseed oil, syrup, pecans and cinnamon.

Drizzle over baked or mashed sweet potato or squash, steamed parsnips, carrots or Brussels sprouts, scones or popcorn.

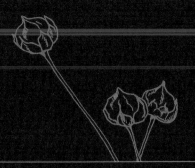

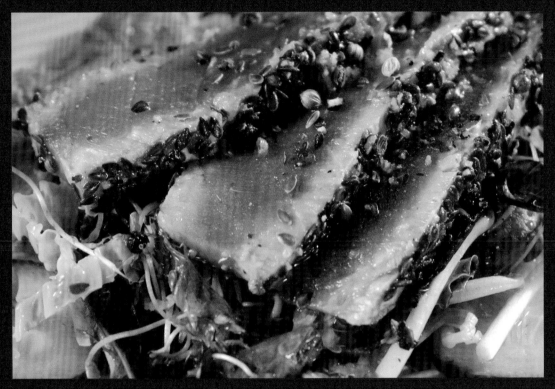

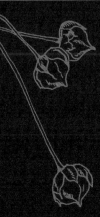

Pictured: *Pan-Seared Tuna* (page 146)

Main Dishes

Mealtimes provide special opportunities for families and friends to not only share food, but also to come together and enjoy each other's company. By incorporating flax in your meals, eating becomes something you can definitely feel good about.

This chapter features classic comfort dishes like Chicken with Herb Stuffing or Meat Loaf, old favourites like Lasagna and vegetarian delights such as Brown Rice–Stuffed Portobello Mushrooms. Look no further than these versatile family- and company-pleasing entrées inspired by our family and friends. Better yet, create your own!

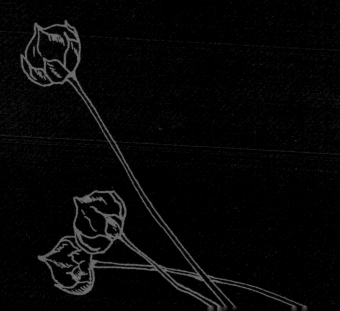

THREE-BEAN CHILI

Flax Fact: Flaxseed is considered one of the most nutritious plant proteins. Its protein profile is similar to that of the soybean. This is particularly significant to vegetarians relying on plant sources to meet their daily protein requirements.

1 lb (500 g) lean ground beef
2 Tbsp (25 mL) flaxseed oil
1½ cups (375 mL) chopped onion
1½ cups (375 mL) chopped green
   bell pepper
1 cup (250 mL) chopped celery
2 Tbsp (25 mL) chili powder
1 tsp (5 mL) ground cumin
4 cloves garlic, minced
1 Tbsp (15 mL) flaxseed oil
28 oz (796 mL) can whole tomatoes,
   chopped

19 oz (540 mL) can red kidney
   beans, rinsed and drained
19 oz (540 mL) can chickpeas,
   rinsed and drained
19 oz (540 mL) can black beans,
   rinsed and drained
1 Tbsp (15 mL) salt
1 tsp (5 mL) black pepper
1 Tbsp (15 mL) whole toasted
   flaxseed per serving

YIELD: 10 cups (2.5 L)

NUTRIENT VALUES PER
SERVING (1 CUP/250 ML)

Calories	382
Protein	22.6 g
Carbohydrates	44.9 g
Fibre	15.8 g
Fat	14.1 g
Saturated	2.8 g
Monounsaturated	3.8 g
Polyunsaturated	5.7 g
Cholesterol	33 mg
Folate	101 mcg
Potassium	646 mg
Sodium	1295 mg

1. In a Dutch oven or large saucepan, break up the ground beef into small pieces.
2. Add the 2 Tbsp (25 mL) flaxseed oil and cook the beef over medium-low heat until no longer pink.
3. Add the onion, bell pepper, celery, chili powder, cumin and garlic. Cook until the onion is tender.
4. Add 1 Tbsp (15 mL) flaxseed oil, tomatoes, kidney beans, chickpeas, black beans, salt and pepper.
5. Bring to a boil, cover and reduce the heat to low. Simmer for 20 minutes.
6. Pour 1 cup (250 mL) of chili into each bowl and sprinkle 1 Tbsp (15 mL) of the flaxseed overtop.

HOME-STYLE MEAT LOAF

2 lb (1 kg) lean ground beef

1 cup (250 mL) skim milk

½ cup (125 mL) ground flaxseed

½ cup (125 mL) dry breadcrumbs

½ cup (125 mL) chopped onion

1 egg, beaten

1 Tbsp (15 mL) Worcestershire sauce

1 tsp (5 mL) black pepper

1 tsp (5 mL) garlic powder

1 tsp (5 mL) dried mustard

½ tsp (2 mL) celery salt

¼ tsp (1 mL) ground thyme

¼ cup (50 mL) ketchup

YIELD: 1 loaf (8 slices)

NUTRIENT VALUES PER
SERVING (1 SLICE)

Calories	375
Protein	27.6 g
Carbohydrates	15.5 g
Fibre	2.9 g
Fat	22.3 g
Saturated	7.2 g
Monounsaturated	8.5 g
Polyunsaturated	3.9 g
Cholesterol	104 mg
Folate	59 mcg
Potassium	598 mg
Sodium	258 mg

1. Preheat the oven to 350°F (180°C).
2. In a large bowl, combine the beef, milk, flaxseed, breadcrumbs, onion, egg, Worcestershire sauce, pepper, garlic powder, mustard, celery salt and thyme. Mix well.
3. Pat the mixture into an ungreased 9- × 5-inch (23 × 12 cm) loaf pan.
4. Spread ketchup overtop the loaf.
5. Bake for 1 to 1½ hours, until no pink remains.
6. Remove from the oven and let stand for 5 minutes.
7. Remove from the pan and place on a platter to serve.

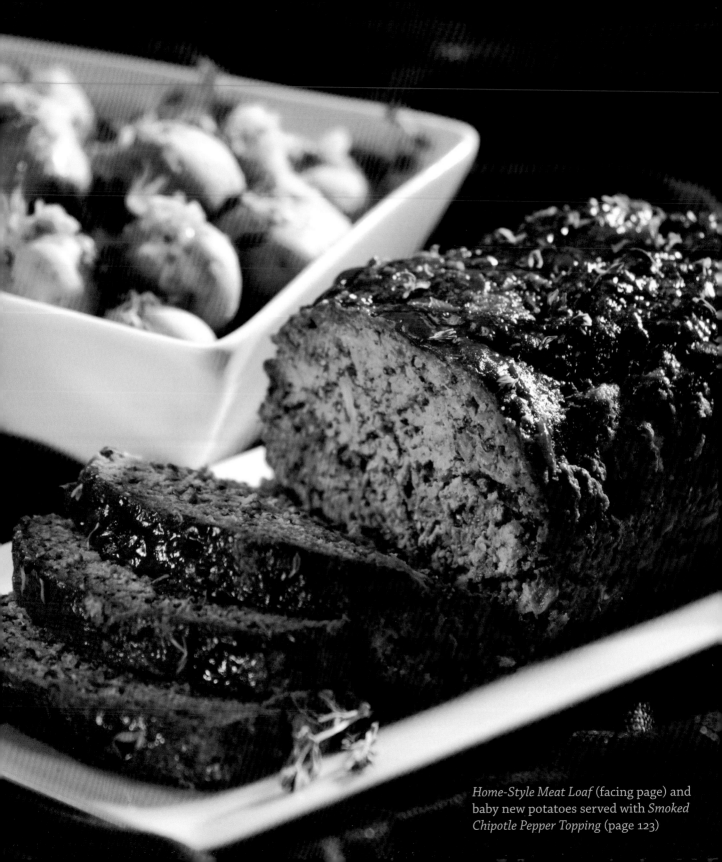

Home-Style Meat Loaf (facing page) and baby new potatoes served with *Smoked Chipotle Pepper Topping* (page 123)

GOLDEN FLAX RAVIOLI

Dough

1½ cups (375 mL) unbleached
   all-purpose flour

¼ cup (50 mL) ground golden flaxseed

1 large egg

¼ cup (50 mL) warm water
   (100 to 110°F/40 to 45°C)

Filling

1 large egg

1 cup (250 mL) partially skimmed
   ricotta cheese

¼ cup (50 mL) grated Parmesan
   cheese

2 Tbsp (25 mL) chopped chives

¼ tsp (1 mL) salt

¼ tsp (1 mL) black pepper

YIELD: 4 servings

NUTRIENT VALUES PER
SERVING (6 RAVIOLI)

Calories	360
Protein	19.5 g
Carbohydrates	42.5 g
Fibre	4.0 g
Fat	13.1 g
Saturated	6.5 g
Monounsaturated	4.0 g
Polyunsaturated	1.8 g
Cholesterol	117 mg
Folate	101 mcg
Potassium	256 mg
Sodium	375 mg

1. For the dough, in a bowl, combine the flour and flaxseed. Mix well.
2. Make a well in the centre of the flour mixture and break the egg into it. Beat the egg with a fork, slowly bringing in the flour.
3. As the dough starts to thicken, work it with your fingers, adding the warm water gradually until all the flour is worked in. Turn out onto a clean work surface.
4. Form the dough into a ball and knead it until smooth, about 2 minutes. Divide the dough into 2 balls.
5. Cover the dough with a bowl and let it rest on the work surface for 15 minutes.
6. On a lightly floured clean work surface, roll 1 ball of dough into a thin 12- × 12-inch (30 × 30 cm) square.
7. For the filling, in a bowl, combine the egg, ricotta, Parmesan cheese, chives, salt and pepper. Mix well.
8. Place 1 rounded tsp (5 mL) of filling in rows at 1-inch (2.5 cm) intervals. Using a pastry brush and water, dampen the dough along the edge and around the mounds.
9. Roll out a second ball of dough as you did with the first. Place it overtop, pressing down firmly around the mounds.
10. With a knife or pasta cutter, cut apart the ravioli. Crimp the edges with a fork.
11. Bring a large pot of salted water to a boil. Add the ravioli. Cook until tender, about 4 minutes. Remove from the water and drain well.

Serve this with your favourite pasta sauce.

SPANISH RICE & CHORIZO SAUSAGE

2 cups (500 mL) water

1 cup (250 mL) brown rice

½ tsp (2 mL) salt

1 lb (500 g) fresh chorizo sausage

1 Tbsp (15 mL) olive oil

¼ cup (50 mL) finely chopped onion

¼ cup (50 mL) finely chopped celery

¼ cup (50 mL) finely chopped green bell pepper

19 oz (540 mL) can diced tomatoes

⅓ cup (75 mL) ground flaxseed

YIELD: 6 servings

NUTRIENT VALUES PER SERVING (1 CUP/250 ML)

Calories	534
Protein	23.0 g
Carbohydrates	33.5 g
Fibre	4.9 g
Fat	35.0 g
Saturated	12.6 g
Monounsaturated	16.7 g
Polyunsaturated	4.0 g
Cholesterol	67 mg
Folate	11 mcg
Potassium	468 mg
Sodium	1260 mg

CHORIZO is a highly seasoned coarsely ground pork sausage that can be bought either fresh or smoked. You can substitute hot or mild Italian sausage if you prefer.

1. In a medium saucepan, boil the water, then add the rice and salt, stirring.
2. Cover, reduce the heat to a simmer and cook until the water is absorbed and the rice is tender, about 45 minutes.
3. While the rice is cooking, remove the sausage meat from its casing.
4. In a skillet over medium to medium-high heat, brown the sausage meat for 2 minutes or until no longer pink. Break up the larger pieces with a wooden spoon. Remove from the pan and drain and discard any fat.
5. Add the olive oil to the skillet.
6. Add the onion, celery and bell pepper. Sauté over medium heat until the vegetables are soft and starting to brown, about 4 minutes.
7. Preheat the oven to 350°F (180°C). Lightly spray a 6-cup (1.5 L) casserole dish with non-stick cooking spray.
8. Combine the cooked rice, sausage meat, sautéed vegetables, diced tomatoes and flaxseed. Mix well.
9. Place the mixture in the casserole dish, cover and bake for 20 minutes.
10. Remove from the oven, stir and let stand, still covered, for 5 minutes before serving.

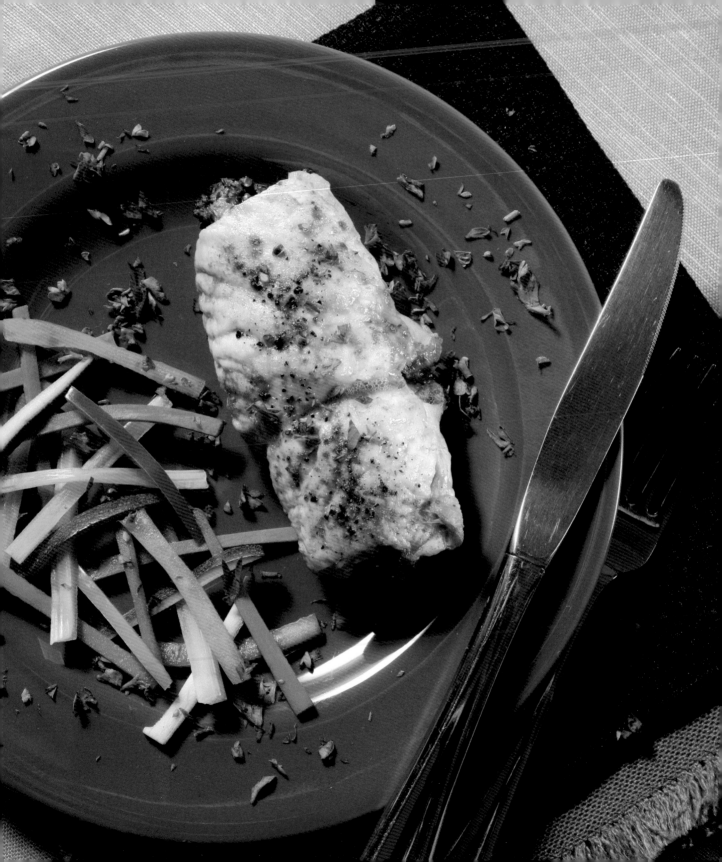

CHICKEN WITH HERB STUFFING

4 boneless, skinless chicken breasts,
    each 6 oz (175 g)
1 Tbsp (15 mL) canola oil
2 tsp (10 mL) minced onion
2 tsp (10 mL) minced red bell pepper
1 Tbsp (15 mL) chopped cran-raisins
2 tsp (10 mL) whole flaxseed
4 slices whole wheat bread, cut into
    ½-inch (1 cm) cubes

2 large eggs
2 Tbsp (25 mL) white wine, apple juice
    or chicken broth
2 Tbsp (25 mL) ground flaxseed
2 tsp (10 mL) chopped fresh parsley
canola oil
salt
black pepper
paprika

YIELD: 4 servings

NUTRIENT VALUES PER
SERVING (1 CHICKEN
BREAST)

Calories	330
Protein	34.5 g
Carbohydrates	17.9 g
Fibre	4.1 g
Fat	13.4 g
Saturated	2.9 g
Monounsaturated	5.8 g
Polyunsaturated	3.4 g
Cholesterol	175 mg
Folate	33 mcg
Potassium	471 mg
Sodium	735 mg

1. Flatten the chicken breasts between 2 sheets of wax paper to ¼-inch (6 mm) thickness.
2. Heat the oil in a skillet over medium-low heat.
3. Add the onion and bell pepper. Sauté for 1 minute.
4. Add the cran-raisins and whole flaxseed. Cook for 2 minutes.
5. Remove the mixture from the heat and let it cool for a few minutes.
6. Preheat the oven to 350°F (180°C). Spray a baking sheet with non-stick cooking spray.
7. In a bowl, combine the bread, eggs, wine, ground flaxseed, parsley and the onion–bell pepper mixture.
8. Season to taste with salt and pepper. Mix well.
9. Spread ½ cup (125 mL) of the stuffing mixture on each breast, then roll them up.
10. Place the chicken rolls on the prepared baking sheet.
11. Lightly brush the tops of the chicken rolls with more canola oil. Sprinkle with salt, pepper and paprika to taste.
12. Bake for 40 to 45 minutes. The rolls should feel firm and bounce back when gently pressed on top.

CHICKEN WITH CRUNCHY FLAX COATING

¼ cup (50 mL) ground toasted golden flaxseed

¼ cup (50 mL) cornmeal

¼ cup (50 mL) coarsely ground corn flakes

2 Tbsp (25 mL) grated Parmesan cheese

½ tsp (2 mL) garlic powder

1 tsp (5 mL) dried parsley flakes

½ tsp (2 mL) salt

¼ tsp (1 mL) black pepper

pinch ground sage

¼ cup (50 mL) butter, melted

6 boneless, skinless chicken breasts, each 4 oz (125 g)

YIELD: 6 servings

NUTRIENT VALUES PER SERVING (1 BREAST WITH 2 TBSP + 1 TSP/30 ML COATING)

Calories	227
Protein	25.1 g
Carbohydrates	8.1 g
Fibre	1.8 g
Fat	9.9 g
Saturated	4.7 g
Monounsaturated	0.8 g
Polyunsaturated	1.7 g
Cholesterol	76 mg
Folate	31 mcg
Potassium	315 mg
Sodium	282 mg

1. In a bowl, combine the flaxseed, cornmeal, corn flakes, cheese, garlic powder, parsley, salt, pepper and sage. Store in an airtight container until ready to use.
2. Preheat the oven to 400°F (200°C).
3. Pour the melted butter into a shallow pan.
4. Dip each chicken breast in the melted butter. Roll in the coating mixture and evenly coat all sides.
5. Place the chicken in a casserole dish. Bake for 18 to 24 minutes.

You can substitute the chicken with pork cutlets (cook for approximately 12 minutes).

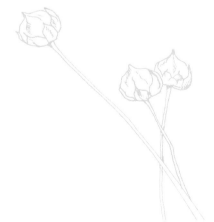

OVEN-FRIED CHICKEN

1 egg, beaten

3 Tbsp (45 mL) skim milk

½ cup (125 mL) ground flaxseed

½ cup (125 mL) finely crushed
   unsalted crackers

1 Tbsp (15 mL) dried parsley flakes

1 tsp (5 mL) paprika

1 tsp (5 mL) chili powder

1 tsp (5 mL) garlic powder

1 tsp (5 mL) seasoned salt

¼ tsp (1 mL) black pepper

2 to 3 lb (1 to 1.5 kg) chicken pieces

YIELD: 6 servings

NUTRIENT VALUES PER
SERVING (1 TO 2 PIECES)

Calories	267
Protein	23.9 g
Carbohydrates	10.1 g
Fibre	3.5 g
Fat	14.7 g
Saturated	4.0 g
Monounsaturated	4.0 g
Polyunsaturated	5.4 g
Cholesterol	107 mg
Folate	67 mcg
Potassium	627 mg
Sodium	147 mg

1. Preheat the oven to 350°F (180°C). Spray a 15- × 10- × ¾-inch (40 × 25 × 2 cm) baking pan with non-stick cooking spray.
2. In a small bowl, combine the egg and milk.
3. In a shallow container, combine the flaxseed, cracker crumbs, parsley, paprika, chili powder, garlic powder, seasoned salt and pepper.
4. Skin the chicken if necessary, rinse it with water and pat it dry.
5. Dip the chicken pieces into the egg mixture, then coat them evenly with the crumb mixture.
6. Place the chicken on the prepared pan so the pieces don't touch.
7. Bake for 45 minutes or until the chicken is tender and no longer pink. Do not turn the chicken pieces while they bake.

CHICKEN WITH BOURBON

¼ cup (50 mL) cornmeal or fine
　dry breadcrumbs

¼ cup (50 mL) whole flaxseed

2 Tbsp (25 mL) unbleached
　all-purpose flour

1 tsp (5 mL) Creole or Cajun
　seasoning

4 boneless, skinless chicken breasts,
　each 4 oz (125 g)

2 Tbsp (25 mL) canola oil

1 Tbsp (15 mL) minced onion

1 Tbsp (15 mL) chopped fresh thyme

1 Tbsp (15 mL) chopped fresh parsley

1 clove garlic, minced

salt

black pepper

⅓ cup (75 mL) chicken stock

¼ cup (50 mL) bourbon or whiskey

2 tsp (10 mL) brown sugar

½ tsp (2 mL) cornstarch

YIELD: 4 servings

NUTRIENT VALUES PER
SERVING (1 BREAST WITH
2 TBSP/25 ML SAUCE)

Calories	303
Protein	30.3 g
Carbohydrates	13.7 g
Fibre	3.4 g
Fat	11.5 g
Saturated	2.5 g
Monounsaturated	5.0 g
Polyunsaturated	3.3 g
Cholesterol	69 mg
Folate	15 mcg
Potassium	406 mg
Sodium	276 mg

1. Preheat the oven to 350°F (180°C).

2. In a bowl, combine the cornmeal, flaxseed, flour and Creole seasoning.

3. Moisten the chicken breasts with water.

4. Coat the chicken breasts evenly with the crumb mixture.

5. In a 10-inch (25 cm) non-stick skillet, heat the oil over medium to medium-high heat. Sear the chicken for 2½ minutes on each side.

6. Remove the chicken from the skillet and finish baking it in the oven until done, about 25 minutes.

7. Meanwhile, in the same skillet, over medium-high heat, sauté the onion until soft, about 2 minutes. Add the thyme, parsley, garlic, salt and pepper. Stir.

8. Add the chicken stock and bourbon and heat for about 30 seconds.

9. Add the brown sugar and cornstarch. Stir the mixture and bring it to a boil. Remove from the heat.

10. Spoon the sauce over each breast before serving.

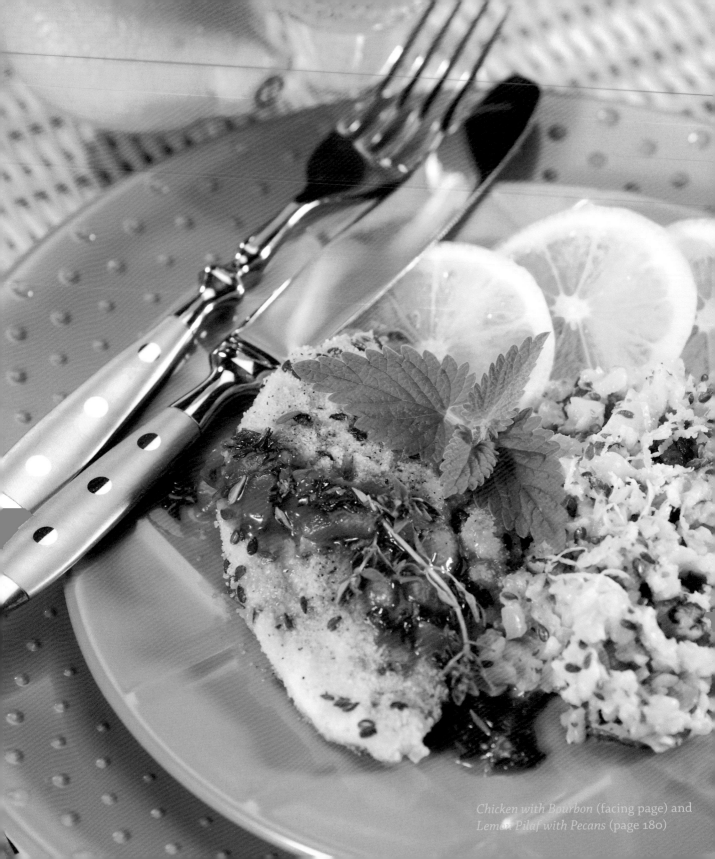

Chicken with Bourbon (facing page) and
Lemon Pilaf with Pecans (page 180)

COUNTRY-STYLE LASAGNA

Meat sauce

1 lb (500 g) lean ground beef

1 cup (250 mL) chopped onion

⅓ cup (75 mL) chopped green bell
  pepper

2 cloves garlic, minced

14 oz (398 mL) can diced tomatoes

14 oz (398 mL) can tomato sauce

5½ oz (156 mL) can tomato paste

½ cup (125 mL) water

2 tsp (10 mL) crushed dried basil

2 tsp (10 mL) crushed dried oregano

¼ tsp (1 mL) crushed red chili flakes

¼ tsp (1 mL) black pepper

¼ tsp (1 mL) ground cinnamon

¼ cup (50 mL) ground flaxseed

Pasta

6 uncooked whole wheat lasagna
  noodles

Filling

8 oz (250 g) package frozen chopped
  spinach, thawed and squeezed dry

16 oz (500 g) carton 1% cream-style
  cottage cheese

¼ cup (50 mL) grated light Parmesan
  cheese

¼ cup (50 mL) chopped fresh parsley

¼ cup (50 mL) ground flaxseed

pinch ground nutmeg

1 egg, beaten

2 cups (500 mL) grated partly skimmed
  mozzarella cheese

grated light Parmesan cheese (optional)

YIELD: 8 servings

NUTRIENT VALUES PER
SERVING (1 PIECE)

Calories	485
Protein	42.7 g
Carbohydrates	35.1 g
Fibre	7.5 g
Fat	21.8 g
Saturated	9.8 g
Monounsaturated	8.0 g
Polyunsaturated	2.2 g
Cholesterol	93 mg
Folate	75 mcg
Potassium	1086 mg
Sodium	1004 mg

1. In a large saucepan or Dutch oven over medium to medium-high heat, cook the ground beef, onion, bell pepper and garlic until the beef is brown, about 8 minutes. Drain off and discard any fat.

2. Stir in the diced tomatoes with the juice, tomato sauce, tomato paste, water, basil, oregano, chili flakes, pepper and cinnamon. Bring to a boil.

3. Reduce the heat, cover and simmer for 15 minutes, stirring occasionally.

4. Remove from the heat and stir in ¼ cup (50 mL) flaxseed.

5. Lay the lasagna noodles in a 9- × 12-inch (23 cm × 30 cm) casserole dish. Pour boiling water over to completely cover the noodles and soak them for 15 minutes to soften. Drain them in a colander and set them aside until needed. Dry the casserole dish.

6. Preheat the oven to 350°F (180°C).

7. In a bowl, combine the spinach, cottage cheese, Parmesan cheese, parsley, ¼ cup (50 mL) flaxseed, nutmeg and egg.

8. Spread 1 cup (250 mL) of the meat sauce on the bottom of the casserole dish.

9. Layer 3 noodles on top.

10. Spread half the cheese-spinach filling on top.

11. Top with half the remaining meat sauce and 1 cup (250 mL) of the grated mozzarella cheese.

12. Repeat the noodles, cheese-spinach and meat sauce layers.

13. Bake for 40 to 50 minutes or until the lasagna is bubbling all around the edges and hot in the middle.

14. Top with the remaining mozzarella cheese and bake for another 5 minutes.

15. Remove from the oven and let stand for 10 minutes before cutting into 8 pieces.

16. Serve with extra grated Parmesan cheese (if desired).

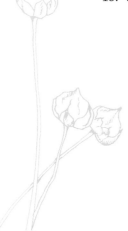

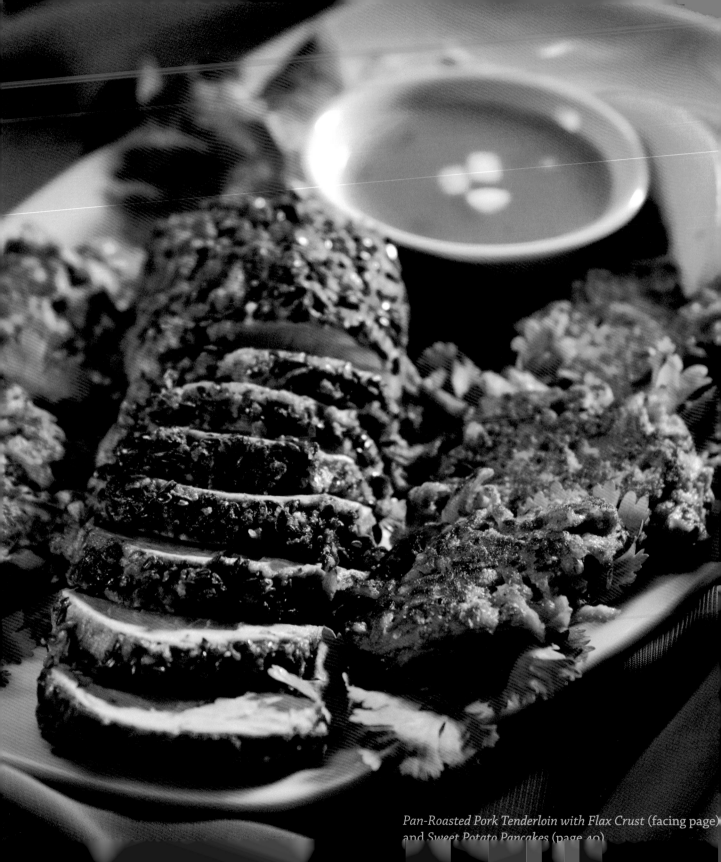

Pan-Roasted Pork Tenderloin with Flax Crust (facing page) and *Sweet Potato Pancakes* (page 40)

PAN-ROASTED PORK TENDERLOIN
WITH FLAX CRUST

⅓ cup (75 mL) canola oil

2 Tbsp (25 mL) balsamic vinegar

1 clove garlic, minced

1 Tbsp (15 mL) chopped fresh herbs
(thyme, oregano, basil, parsley, etc.)

1 lb (500 g) pork tenderloin

½ cup (125 mL) whole flaxseed

2 Tbsp (25 mL) unbleached
all-purpose flour

1 Tbsp (15 mL) chili powder

1½ tsp (7 mL) cumin seeds, toasted
and ground (see sidebar)

salt

black pepper

YIELD: 4 servings

NUTRIENT VALUES PER
SERVING (6 SLICES)

Calories	458
Protein	31.4 g
Carbohydrates	13.0 g
Fibre	7.6 g
Fat	34.8 g
Saturated	7.8 g
Monounsaturated	16.3 g
Polyunsaturated	9.1 g
Cholesterol	83 mg
Folate	13 mcg
Potassium	673 mg
Sodium	333 mg

TO TOAST CUMIN SEEDS, heat them in a small skillet over medium heat for 1½ minutes or until the seeds turn a darker shade and are fragrant. They burn easily, so keep a close eye on them. Grind them with a blunt wooden or metal object.

1. In a bowl, combine the oil, vinegar, garlic and herbs. Add the tenderloin to the bowl and turn it to coat evenly.

2. Cover and refrigerate the tenderloin for 4 to 6 hours.

3. Lay a sheet of wax paper on a clean work surface. Combine the flaxseed, flour, chili powder, cumin, and salt and pepper to taste on the wax paper.

4. Preheat the oven to 375°F (190°C).

5. Drain the tenderloin and roll it in the flaxseed mixture to coat it evenly.

6. Heat a cast iron skillet (or any ovenproof skillet) over medium-high heat. Sear the tenderloin on all sides until browned, about 3 minutes.

7. Place the pan in the oven and roast the tenderloin uncovered until the internal temperature reaches 160°F (71°C), about 25 minutes.

8. Remove the tenderloin from the oven. Place it on a cutting board and let it rest for 5 minutes.

9. Cut the tenderloin crosswise into 24 thin slices.

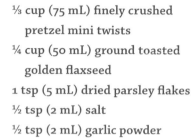

PORK CUTLETS WITH FLAX PRETZEL COATING

⅓ cup (75 mL) finely crushed
  pretzel mini twists

¼ cup (50 mL) ground toasted
  golden flaxseed

1 tsp (5 mL) dried parsley flakes

½ tsp (2 mL) salt

½ tsp (2 mL) garlic powder

¼ cup (50 mL) butter

3 Tbsp (45 mL) prepared mustard

4 drops hot sauce

1 Tbsp (15 mL) unbleached
  all-purpose flour

4 pork cutlets, each 4 oz (125 g)

YIELD: 4 servings

NUTRIENT VALUES PER
SERVING (1 PORK CUTLET
WITH 2 TBSP + 1 TSP/
30 ML) COATING)

Calories	298
Protein	24.1 g
Carbohydrates	8.4 g
Fibre	2.5 g
Fat	18.6 g
Saturated	8.3 g
Monounsaturated	5.9 g
Polyunsaturated	3.1 g
Cholesterol	85 mg
Folate	18 mcg
Potassium	477 mg
Sodium	562 mg

1. In a bowl, combine the ground pretzels, flaxseed, parsley, salt and garlic powder.
2. Preheat the oven to 400°F (200°C).
3. Melt the butter in a small saucepan. Whisk in the mustard and hot sauce and transfer the mixture into a shallow pan.
4. Dip the pork cutlets into the butter mixture to coat both sides, then roll in the coating mixture to coat evenly.
5. Place the cutlets on a baking pan. Bake for approximately 12 minutes.

Store any extra unused coating in an airtight container in the freezer. You can substitute the pork cutlets with chicken breasts. If using chicken, bake for 18 to 24 minutes.

HAM 'N' SWISS MEAL-IN-A-LOAF

3 cups (750 mL) unbleached
   all-purpose flour

2 Tbsp (25 mL) granulated sugar

½ tsp (2 mL) salt

¼ cup (50 mL) whole flaxseed

1 Tbsp (15 mL) quick-rising yeast

1 cup (250 mL) water

¼ cup (50 mL) dried mustard

2 Tbsp (25 mL) margarine

1 egg, beaten, for brushing (optional)

1½ cups (375 mL) diced cooked ham

1 cup (250 mL) shredded Swiss cheese

½ cup (125 mL) diced dill pickles

YIELD: 1 loaf (14 slices)

NUTRIENT VALUES PER
SERVING (1 SLICE)

Calories	211
Protein	10.9 g
Carbohydrates	25.4 g
Fibre	1.8 g
Fat	6.6 g
Saturated	2.2 g
Monounsaturated	1.8 g
Polyunsaturated	1.6 g
Cholesterol	18 mg
Folate	38 mcg
Potassium	162 mg
Sodium	387 mg

1. Prepare a baking sheet by spraying it with non-stick cooking spray.
2. In a large bowl, combine 2 cups (500 mL) of the flour with the sugar, salt, flax-seed and yeast.
3. Heat the water, mustard and margarine in a small saucepan over low heat until the liquid is hot to the touch, about 120 to 130°F (50 to 55°C). Stir this into the flour mixture.
4. Gradually add enough of the reserved flour to make a soft, non-sticky dough. Knead the dough for 4 minutes, then roll it into a 14- × 12-inch (35 × 30 cm) rectangle.
5. Sprinkle the ham, cheese and pickles down the centre of the dough.
6. Make cuts from the filling to the edge of the dough at 1-inch (2.5 cm) intervals.
7. Bring the strips together and overlap them in a braid-like design, encasing the filling in the dough. Place this on the prepared baking sheet and let it rest in a warm, draft-free place for 15 minutes.
8. Preheat the oven to 375°F (190°C).
9. Brush the top of the dough with the egg (if using).
10. Bake for 25 minutes or until golden.
11. Cool on a rack.

PAN-SEARED TUNA

2 Tbsp (25 mL) fresh orange juice

2 Tbsp (25 mL) rice wine vinegar

1 tsp (5 mL) freshly grated ginger

½ tsp (2 mL) curry paste
(see sidebar)

3 Tbsp (45 mL) flaxseed oil

1 Tbsp (15 mL) sesame oil

black pepper

2 Tbsp (25 mL) whole flaxseed

1 Tbsp (15 mL) assorted peppercorns,
cracked

1 tsp (5 mL) coarse sea salt

12 oz (375 g) fresh tuna (ahi or yellow
fin), 1 inch (2.5 cm) thick

2 Tbsp (25 mL) canola oil

twenty-four ⅛-inch (3 mm) slices
English cucumber

½ cup (125 mL) assorted sprouts
(alfalfa, radish, etc.)
or 1 cup (250 mL) bean sprouts

2 cups (500 mL) packed seasonal greens
(spring or mesclun mix may be used)

YIELD: 4 servings

NUTRIENT VALUES PER
SERVING (3 OZ/90 G
TUNA, ½ CUP/125 ML
GREENS AND 2 TBSP/
25 ML VINAIGRETTE)

Calories	313
Protein	23.8 g
Carbohydrates	4.7 g
Fibre	2.4 g
Fat	22.8 g
Saturated	3.0 g
Monounsaturated	7.4 g
Polyunsaturated	11.3 g
Cholesterol	42 mg
Folate	32 mcg
Potassium	594 mg
Sodium	678 mg

CURRY PASTE ranges in
strength from mild to hot
and is found in the ethnic
section of large supermarkets. You can also use 1 tsp
(5 mL) curry powder instead.

1. In a small bowl, stir together the orange juice, vinegar, ginger and curry paste.
2. Slowly whisk in the flaxseed and sesame oils. Season to taste with pepper.
3. In another bowl, combine the flaxseed, peppercorns and sea salt. Coat the tuna evenly with the flaxseed mixture.
4. Heat a non-stick pan over medium-high heat.
5. Add the canola oil.
6. Sear the tuna for 30 seconds on each side for rare or up to 1½ minutes on each side for medium. Do not overcook.
7. Remove the tuna from the pan and let it rest on a cutting board for 2 minutes before slicing.
8. Arrange 6 cucumber slices on each plate to form a circle 6 inches (15 cm) in diameter.
9. Build a sprout-and-greens salad inside each cucumber circle.
10. Slice the tuna into 20 slices (5 slices per serving) and place them on top of the greens.
11. Drizzle 2 Tbsp (25 mL) of the vinaigrette over each serving of tuna and greens.

Serve with Flax Scones (page 23) if desired.

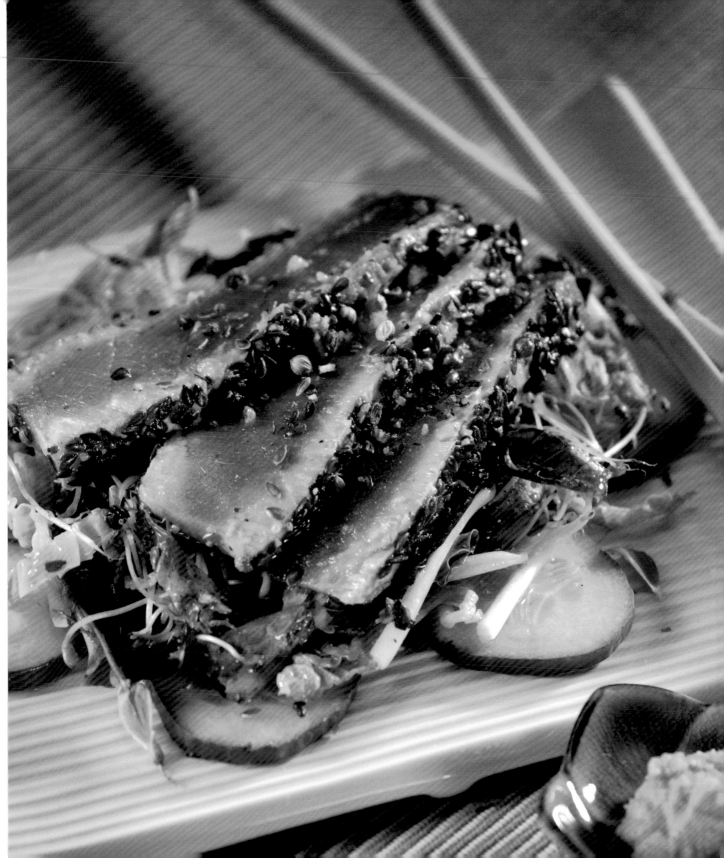

VEGETABLE, RICE & BEAN PIE

Flax Fact: Flax is one of the best plant sources of lignans, natural antioxidants that may reduce the activity of cell-damaging free radicals, slow the aging process, and increase overall wellness. Flaxseed provides up to 700 times more lignans than whole grains or legumes.

Crust

2 cups (500 mL) cooked white rice

1 cup (250 mL) grated mozzarella
cheese

1 egg, beaten

Filling

1 Tbsp (15 mL) olive oil

1 cup (250 mL) chopped onion

½ cup (125 mL) chopped celery

½ cup (125 mL) diced red bell pepper

½ cup (125 mL) diced green bell pepper

1 tsp (5 mL) ground cumin

3 garlic cloves, minced

¼ tsp (1 mL) diced green jalapeño
pepper

19 oz (540 mL) can mixed beans,
rinsed and drained

1½ cups (375 mL) frozen cubed
hash browns

¾ cup (175 mL) old-fashioned
rolled oats

¾ cup (175 mL) ground flaxseed

⅓ cup (75 mL) barbecue sauce

⅓ cup (75 mL) ketchup

⅓ cup (75 mL) chopped fresh cilantro

1 Tbsp (15 mL) tomato paste

1 Tbsp (15 mL) prepared mustard

1½ tsp (7 mL) salt

½ tsp (2 mL) black pepper

¼ tsp (1 mL) crushed red chili flakes

¼ cup (50 mL) barbecue sauce

⅓ cup (75 mL) grated mozzarella cheese

1. Preheat the oven to 350°F (180°C). Spray a 9-inch (23 cm) deep-dish pie plate with non-stick cooking spray.
2. In a bowl, combine the rice, cheese and egg. Mix well and press the mixture into the prepared pie plate.
3. Heat the oil in a large skillet.
4. Sauté the onion, celery, red and green bell peppers, cumin, garlic and jalapeño pepper for 3 minutes.
5. Add the beans and hash browns. Cook over low heat for 5 minutes.
6. Add the oats and mix thoroughly. Turn the mixture into the rice crust and bake for 45 minutes.

YIELD: one 9-inch
(23 cm) pie (12 slices)

NUTRIENT VALUES PER
SERVING (1 SLICE)

Calories	262
Protein	10.8 g
Carbohydrates	38.6 g
Fibre	7.2 g
Fat	8.7 g
Saturated	3.6 g
Monounsaturated	3.0 g
Polyunsaturated	1.7 g
Cholesterol	26 mg
Folate	83 mcg
Potassium	461 mg
Sodium	694 mg

7. In a bowl, combine the flaxseed, barbecue sauce, ketchup, cilantro, tomato paste, mustard, salt, pepper and chili flakes. Set aside.

8. Remove the pie from the oven.

9. Reduce the oven temperature to 325°F (160°C).

10. Brush the barbecue sauce over the pie and sprinkle it with the cheese.

11. Return the pie to the oven and bake for 15 minutes longer. Remove it from the oven and let it sit for 5 minutes. Slice and serve.

VEGGIE CALZONES

Dough

1½ cups (375 mL) unbleached
   all-purpose flour

½ cup (125 mL) ground flaxseed

1 tsp (5 mL) granulated sugar

1 tsp (5 mL) salt

one 8 g package (2¼ tsp/11 mL)
   quick-rising yeast

½ cup (125 mL) very warm water
   (120 to 130°F/50 to 55°C)

2 Tbsp (25 mL) canola oil

⅓ cup (75 mL) 1% milk

Filling

1 cup (250 mL) chopped mushrooms

¾ cup (175 mL) tomato sauce

½ cup (125 mL) grated partially
   skimmed mozzarella cheese

½ cup (125 mL) pineapple tidbits,
   well drained

¼ cup (50 mL) finely chopped onion

¼ cup (50 mL) finely chopped green
   bell pepper

2 Tbsp (25 mL) grated Parmesan cheese

2 Tbsp (25 mL) ground flaxseed

1 tsp (5 mL) crushed dried oregano

1 tsp (5 mL) crushed dried basil

1 clove garlic, crushed

1 Tbsp (15 mL) cornmeal

canola oil

YIELD: 8 calzones

NUTRIENT VALUES PER
SERVING (1 CALZONE)

Calories	207
Protein	8.4 g
Carbohydrates	26.9 g
Fibre	4.6 g
Fat	9.0 g
Saturated	3.0 g
Monounsaturated	3.4 g
Polyunsaturated	2.3 g
Cholesterol	6 mg
Folate	63 mcg
Potassium	284 mg
Sodium	501 mg

1. For the dough, in a large bowl, combine the flour, flaxseed, sugar, salt and yeast. Add the water and oil. Stir well with a fork.

2. Gradually add enough milk until the dough forms a ball. Knead well for 2 minutes.

3. Place the dough on a lightly floured clean work surface, cover with a bowl and let rest for 10 minutes.

4. For the filling, in a medium bowl, mix together the mushrooms, tomato sauce, mozzarella cheese, pineapple, onion, bell pepper, Parmesan cheese, flaxseed, oregano, basil and garlic.

5. Preheat the oven to 450°F (230°C). Sprinkle a baking sheet with cornmeal.

6. Divide the dough into 8 equal portions. Roll each piece into a 5-inch (12 cm) circle.

7. In the centre of each circle, place ¼ cup (50 mL) of filling.

Continued on page 154 . . .

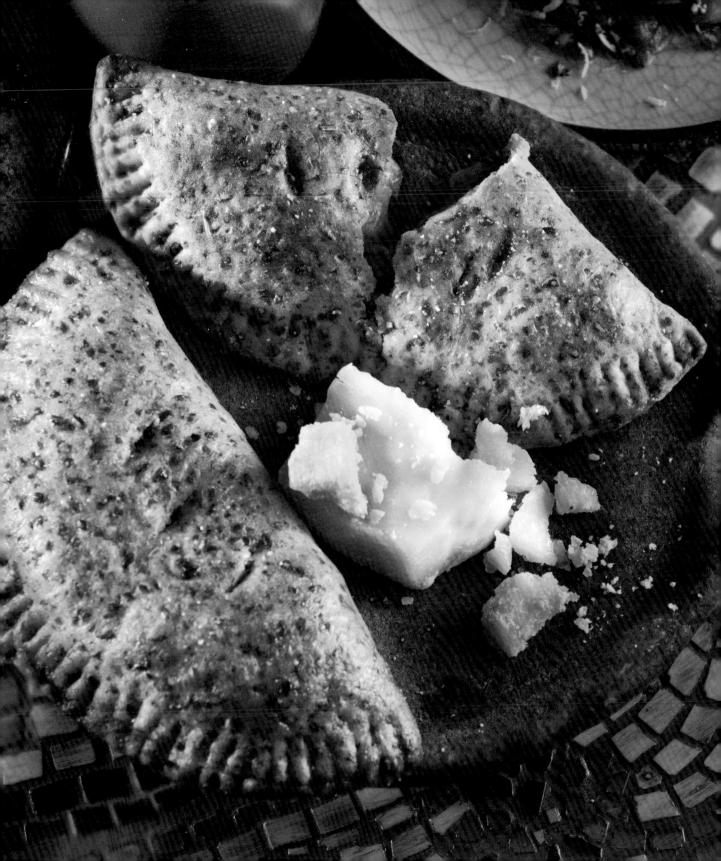

VEGGIE CALZONES *(Continued)* . . .

8. Fold the dough over to form a half-circle. Crimp the edges well. With a fork or the point of a sharp knife, poke holes in the top of each calzone to allow steam to escape.

9. Place the calzones 2 inches (5 cm) apart on the prepared baking sheet. Lightly brush the tops with canola oil.

10. Bake for 15 to 20 minutes or until golden.

11. Remove from the oven and let cool for 10 minutes before eating.

The calzones can be completely cooled, wrapped and frozen. Reheat frozen calzones on high power in the microwave for about 2 minutes.

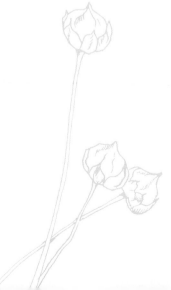

VEGETARIAN RAGOUT

¼ cup (50 mL) flaxseed oil

2 cups (500 mL) chopped zucchini

1½ cups (375 mL) chopped onion

1½ cups (375 mL) chopped carrot

1 cup (250 mL) chopped green bell
pepper

1 cup (250 mL) chopped celery

2 cloves garlic, minced

28 oz (796 mL) can whole tomatoes,
chopped

2 tsp (10 mL) salt

1 tsp (5 mL) ground cumin

1 tsp (5 mL) dried rosemary

½ tsp (2 mL) ground thyme

½ tsp (2 mL) ground coriander

¼ tsp (1 mL) ground nutmeg

¼ tsp (1 mL) ground cinnamon

19 oz (540 mL) can romano beans,
rinsed and drained

19 oz (540 mL) can kidney beans, rinsed
and drained

19 oz (540 mL) can chickpeas, rinsed
and drained

1 Tbsp (15 mL) whole toasted flaxseed
per serving

YIELD: 11 cups (2.75 L)

NUTRIENT VALUES PER
SERVING (1 CUP/250 ML)

Calories	304
Protein	13.2 g
Carbohydrates	44.4 g
Fibre	16.3 g
Fat	9.5 g
Saturated	0.9 g
Monounsaturated	1.7 g
Polyunsaturated	6.0 g
Cholesterol	0 mg
Folate	176 mcg
Potassium	522 mg
Sodium	705 mg

1. In a Dutch oven or large saucepan, heat the flaxseed oil over medium-low heat.
2. Add the zucchini, onion, carrot, green bell pepper, celery and garlic. Sauté for
   4 minutes.
3. Add the tomatoes, salt, cumin, rosemary, thyme, coriander, nutmeg and
   cinnamon. Heat to a boil. Reduce the heat, cover and simmer for 20 minutes,
   stirring occasionally.
4. Add the beans and chickpeas. Cook gently until heated through.
5. Serve over couscous or brown rice and sprinkle each serving with flaxseed.

BROWN RICE–STUFFED PORTOBELLO MUSHROOMS

2 cups (500 mL) cooked brown rice

¼ cup (50 mL) whole flaxseed

2 eggs

½ cup (125 mL) 2% milk

1 cup (250 mL) grated cheddar
cheese

½ cup (125 mL) finely chopped onion

½ cup (125 mL) finely chopped celery

1 tsp (5 mL) crushed dried basil

½ tsp (2 mL) seasoned salt

pinch black pepper

6 portobello mushrooms, 4 inches
(10 cm) in diameter

6 tsp (30 mL) flaxseed oil

6 tsp (30 mL) balsamic vinegar

YIELD: 6 servings

NUTRIENT VALUES PER
SERVING (1 MUSHROOM)

Calories	288
Protein	12.6 g
Carbohydrates	24.6 g
Fibre	5.5 g
Fat	16.3 g
Saturated	5.5 g
Monounsaturated	4.1 g
Polyunsaturated	5.6 g
Cholesterol	83 mg
Folate	51 mcg
Potassium	612 mg
Sodium	217 mg

1. Preheat the oven to 350°F (180°C). Spray two 9-inch (23 cm) pie plates with non-stick cooking spray.
2. In a medium bowl, combine the cooked brown rice and flaxseed.
3. Add the egg and milk and beat the mix with a fork until well mixed.
4. Add the cheese, onion, celery, basil, salt and pepper.
5. Remove the stems from the mushroom caps and chop them finely. Add the chopped stems to the rice mixture.
6. Place the mushroom caps, tops down, in the prepared pie plates.
7. Evenly divide the rice mixture between the mushroom caps.
8. Loosely cover the pie plates with aluminum foil.
9. Bake the mushrooms for 40 to 45 minutes or until the mixture is set.
10. Let cool in the pan for 5 minutes.
11. Drizzle the bottom of each serving plate with 1 tsp (5 mL) each of flaxseed oil and balsamic vinegar.
12. Place a mushroom cap on each plate and serve.

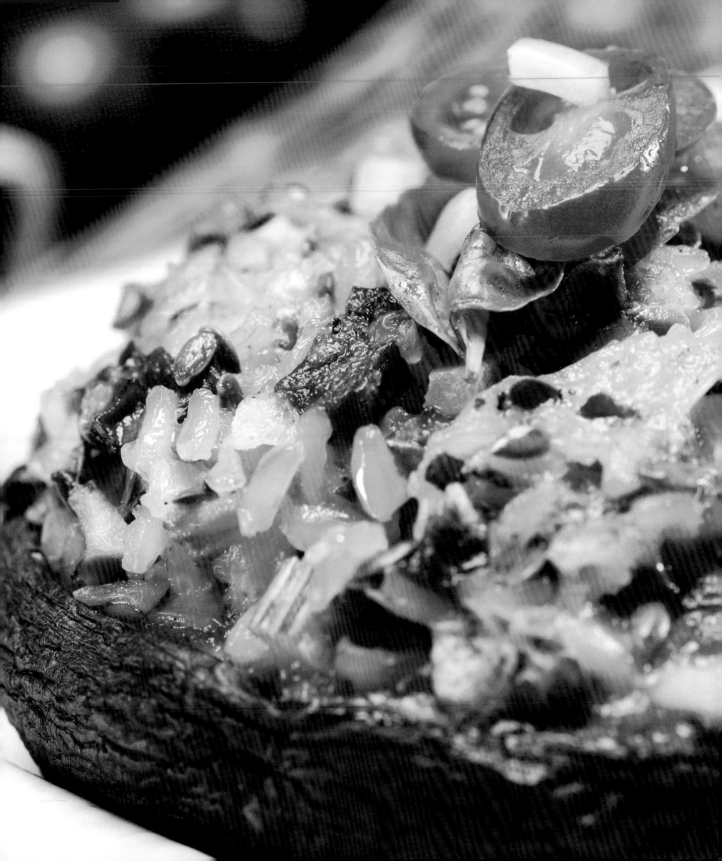

BAKED ITALIAN SANDWICHES

Filling

3 Italian sausages (hot or mild), casing removed

¼ cup (50 mL) diced green bell pepper

¼ cup (50 mL) diced onion

2 Tbsp (25 mL) tomato paste

2 Tbsp (25 mL) ground flaxseed

Dough

¾ cup (175 mL) unbleached all-purpose flour

½ cup (125 mL) cornmeal

¼ cup (50 mL) ground flaxseed

2 Tbsp (25 mL) grated Parmesan cheese

2 tsp (10 mL) baking powder

1 tsp (5 mL) crushed dried oregano

½ tsp (2 mL) salt

1 clove garlic, minced

2 Tbsp (25 mL) olive oil

½ cup (125 mL) 1% milk

YIELD: 7 sandwiches

NUTRIENT VALUES PER SERVING (1 SANDWICH)

Calories	266
Protein	11.1 g
Carbohydrates	23.3 g
Fibre	3.8 g
Fat	15.5 g
Saturated	4.9 g
Monounsaturated	7.4 g
Polyunsaturated	2.4 g
Cholesterol	25 mg
Folate	48 mcg
Potassium	296 mg
Sodium	565 mg

1. In a non-stick skillet over medium heat, cook the sausage meat, bell pepper and onion until the meat is no longer pink, about 6 minutes. Drain off and discard the fat.

2. Stir in the tomato paste and flaxseed. Let the mixture cool while you make the dough.

3. Preheat the oven to 450°F (230°C).

4. For the dough, in a medium bowl, combine the flour, cornmeal, flaxseed, Parmesan cheese, baking powder, oregano, salt and garlic. Mix well.

5. Drizzle the olive oil over the flour mixture and stir well. Mix this with your fingers until the mixture resembles coarse crumbs.

6. Add the milk, stirring only until the ingredients are dampened. Add a little more milk if needed to make a soft dough.

7. Turn the dough out onto a clean, well-floured work surface. Knead gently 8 times.

8. Roll the dough into a 14-inch (35 cm) diameter circle ¼ inch (6 mm) thick.

9. Cut six 4½-inch (11 cm) circles. Combine the remaining dough to cut 1 more circle.

10. Spoon 2 Tbsp (25 mL) of filling on half of each circle.

11. Dampen the outside edge with water. Fold half the dough over the filling to meet the other half, forming a semicircle. Seal the edges with a fork.

12. Place the sandwiches on an ungreased baking sheet and bake for 12 to 15 minutes or until lightly browned.

HUMMUS TORTILLA SANDWICH

Hummus

14 oz (398 mL) can chickpeas,
  rinsed and drained

¼ cup (50 mL) water

¼ cup (50 mL) flaxseed, coarsely
  ground or whole

2 tsp (10 mL) olive oil

2 tsp (10 mL) fresh lemon juice

1 tsp (5 mL) sesame oil

1 large clove garlic

¼ tsp (1 mL) salt

¼ tsp (1 mL) ground cumin

pinch cayenne pepper

pinch black pepper

Sandwiches

four 10-inch (25 cm) flax or whole
  wheat tortillas (see page 66)

1 cup (250 mL) coarsely grated
  English cucumber, drained on a
  paper towel

2 Roma tomatoes, diced

alfalfa sprouts

¼ cup (50 mL) ranch dressing

black pepper

YIELD: 4 tortillas

NUTRIENT VALUES PER
SERVING (1 TORTILLA)

Calories	389
Protein	11.3 g
Carbohydrates	51.4 g
Fibre	8.5 g
Fat	16.2 g
Saturated	2.0 g
Monounsaturated	5.4 g
Polyunsaturated	7.2 g
Cholesterol	3 mg
Folate	121 mcg
Potassium	562 mg
Sodium	684 mg

1. In a blender or food processor, blend together the chickpeas, water, flaxseed, olive oil, lemon juice, sesame oil, garlic, salt, cumin, cayenne and black pepper until the mixture has a light, creamy texture.
2. Lay the tortillas flat on a clean work surface.
3. Divide the hummus equally over each tortilla (approximately ⅓ cup/75 mL each). Spread the hummus to within ½ inch (1 cm) of the edge.
4. Lay ¼ cup (50 mL) of cucumber down the centre of each tortilla. Top with a quarter of the diced tomatoes and alfalfa sprouts to taste.
5. Drizzle the sprouts with 1 Tbsp (15 mL) ranch dressing and sprinkle with pepper.
6. Roll up the tortillas, tucking in one end and keeping the other end open.

Serve with olives, marinated peppers or hot pepper sauce if desired.

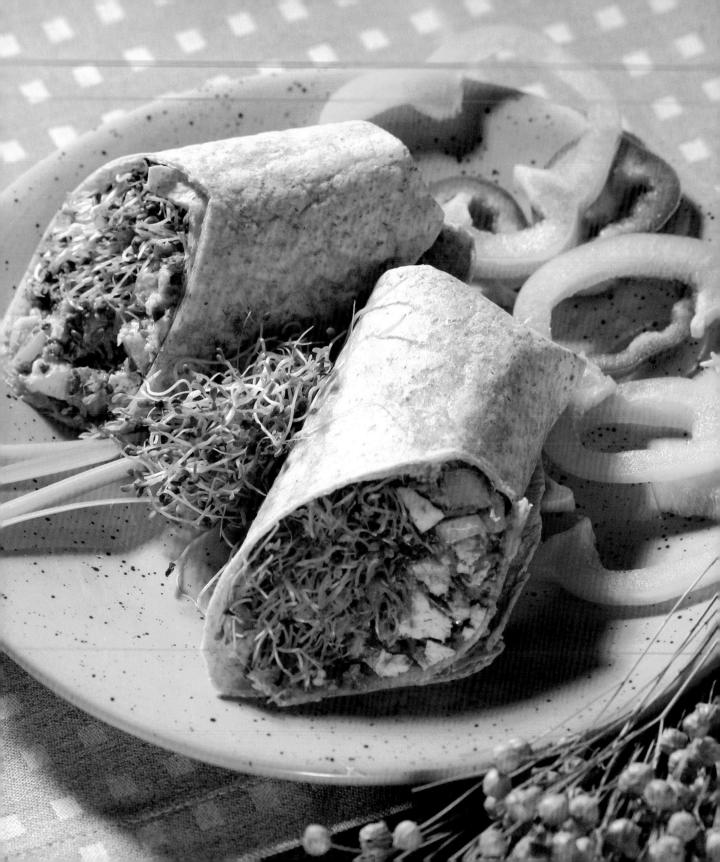

BUFFALO CHICKEN WRAPS

2 cups (500 mL) diced cooked chicken

½ cup (125 mL) shredded carrot

½ cup (125 mL) chopped celery

¼ cup (50 mL) light mayonnaise

2 Tbsp (25 mL) ground flaxseed

2 Tbsp (25 mL) flaxseed oil

2 tsp (10 mL) hot sauce, or to taste

salt

black pepper

four 10-inch (25 cm) flax or whole wheat tortillas (see page 66)

4.2 oz (120 g) package broccoli or alfalfa sprouts

¼ cup (50 mL) crumbled blue cheese

YIELD: 4 wraps

NUTRIENT VALUES PER SERVING (1 WRAP)

Calories	403
Protein	40.6 g
Carbohydrates	26.9 g
Fibre	4.5 g
Fat	17.4 g
Saturated	3.8 g
Monounsaturated	5.3 g
Polyunsaturated	7.1 g
Cholesterol	94 mg
Folate	31 mcg
Potassium	649 mg
Sodium	558 mg

1. In a bowl, combine the chicken, carrot, celery, mayonnaise, ground flaxseed, flaxseed oil, hot sauce, salt and pepper. Mix well.

2. Lay the tortillas on a clean work surface.

3. Place the chicken mixture lengthwise over the lower third of each tortilla.

4. Tear the broccoli sprouts into 4 bunches. Pull apart each bunch slightly to loosen them. Lay the sprouts alongside the filling and sprinkle each wrap with 1 Tbsp (15 mL) of blue cheese.

5. Fold the bottom of the tortilla over the filling and fold the ends in, holding them in place while continuing to roll up the tortilla from the bottom.

6. Wrap each tortilla in plastic wrap or wax paper. Refrigerate for 1 hour to allow the flavours to blend.

7. Slice each roll crosswise on the diagonal before serving.

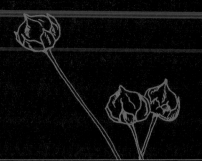
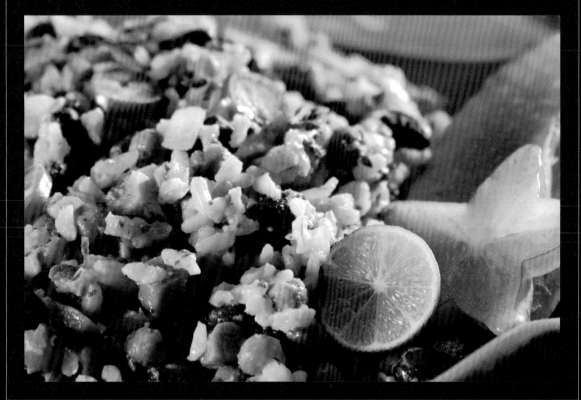
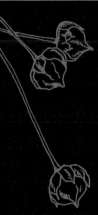

Pictured: *Warm Caribbean Beans & Rice* (page 173)

Side Dishes

Some of the most sophisticated yet simple side dishes combine two of the most ancient and venerable grains—rice and flax. The rice easily absorbs a wide range of flavours, and flaxseed offers a variety of textures (from whole to ground) and high protein content. Together they create fundamentally fabulous vegetarian fare. These dishes are welcome additions to potlucks as they travel and hold well, go with many other flavours and meet a range of tastes. They also hold great appeal for home cooks who like to be organized. Simply make ahead and freeze. Dinner is less of a headache when you can grab one of these side dishes from the freezer.

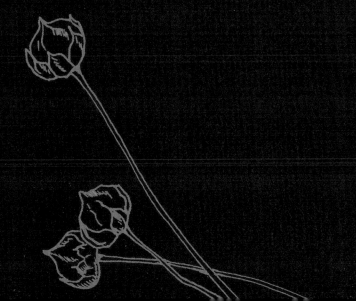

TURNIPS WITH APPLES

Filling

1 to 2 turnips

1 Tbsp (15 mL) butter

2 apples

¼ cup (50 mL) lightly packed
  brown sugar

¼ cup (50 mL) ground flaxseed

pinch ground cinnamon

Topping

⅓ cup (75 mL) unbleached
  all-purpose flour

⅓ cup (75 mL) lightly packed
  brown sugar

3 Tbsp (45 mL) butter

YIELD: 6 servings

NUTRIENT VALUES PER
SERVING (1 CUP/250 ML)

Calories	189
Protein	2.3 g
Carbohydrates	36.9 g
Fibre	3.3 g
Fat	5.2 g
Saturated	2.7 g
Monounsaturated	1.4 g
Polyunsaturated	0.9 g
Cholesterol	9 mg
Folate	19 mcg
Potassium	249 mg
Sodium	66 mg

1. For the filling, peel, dice and boil the turnips until tender.

2. Drain. Add the butter and mash the turnips.

3. Peel, slice and chop the apples.

4. Place the apples in a small bowl and add the ¼ cup (50 mL) brown sugar, flaxseed and cinnamon.

5. Preheat the oven to 350°F (180°C). Spray a casserole dish with non-stick cooking spray.

6. Alternate layers of turnip and apple mixture, beginning and ending with the turnips.

7. For the topping, in a bowl, combine the flour, ⅓ cup (75 mL) brown sugar and butter.

8. Spoon this over the turnip-apple mixture.

9. Bake for 1 hour. Serve.

VEGETABLE STIR-FRY

Vegetables

1 Tbsp (15 mL) canola oil

1 medium onion, cut into thin wedges

½ small zucchini, halved lengthwise and cut into ½-inch (1 cm) slices

1½ cups (375 mL) cauliflower (bite-sized pieces)

1½ cups (375 mL) broccoli (bite-sized pieces)

1 cup (250 mL) sliced fresh mushrooms

½ cup (125 mL) thinly bias-sliced carrots

½ cup (125 mL) green bell pepper strips

½ cup (125 mL) red bell pepper strips

1 Tbsp (15 mL) whole toasted flaxseed

Sauce

2 Tbsp (25 mL) ground toasted flaxseed

1 Tbsp (15 mL) grated fresh ginger

¼ cup (50 mL) vegetable, chicken or beef broth

2 Tbsp (25 mL) soy sauce

1 Tbsp (15 mL) white vinegar

1 tsp (5 mL) granulated sugar

1 clove garlic, minced

YIELD: 4 servings

NUTRIENT VALUES PER SERVING (1½ CUPS/ 375 ML)

Calories	144
Protein	5.5 g
Carbohydrates	18.1 g
Fibre	5.9 g
Fat	7.1 g
Saturated	0.8 g
Monounsaturated	2.2 g
Polyunsaturated	3.7 g
Cholesterol	0 mg
Folate	94 mcg
Potassium	601 mg
Sodium	520 mg

1. Heat the oil in a large skillet.
2. Stir-fry the onion, zucchini, cauliflower, broccoli, mushrooms, carrots and peppers over medium heat for 5 minutes.
3. Cover and cook for another 2 minutes to steam slightly.
4. For the sauce, in a small bowl, combine the ground flaxseed, ginger, broth, soy sauce, vinegar, sugar and garlic.
5. Pour over the vegetables. Cook and stir until bubbly and heated through, about 1 minute.
6. Sprinkle with the 2 Tbsp (25 mL) toasted flaxseed. Serve.

OVEN-FRIED ONION RINGS

½ cup (125 mL) fine dry whole wheat breadcrumbs

2 Tbsp (25 mL) ground flaxseed

1 Tbsp (25 mL) whole flaxseed

2 Tbsp (25 mL) melted butter or margarine

¼ tsp (1 mL) seasoned salt

2 egg whites

2 medium-sized sweet onions, sliced ¼ inch (6 mm) thick (see sidebar)

YIELD: about 30 onion rings

NUTRIENT VALUES PER SERVING (5 ONION RINGS)

Calories	109
Protein	3.7 g
Carbohydrates	11.4 g
Fibre	2.1 g
Fat	6.2 g
Saturated	1.4 g
Monounsaturated	2.4 g
Polyunsaturated	2.2 g
Cholesterol	0 mg
Folate	17 mcg
Potassium	129 mg
Sodium	188 mg

SEPARATE THE ONION SLICES into rings. Use the larger outer rings for this recipe and reserve the smaller inner rings and end pieces for other uses.

1. Preheat the oven to 450°F (230°C). Spray a large baking sheet with non-stick cooking spray.

2. Place the breadcrumbs, ground and whole flaxseed, melted butter and salt on wax paper. Use your fingers to mix them together.

3. In a small bowl, lightly whisk the egg whites until frothy on top.

4. Dip the onion rings in the egg whites, then in the crumb mixture.

5. Arrange the onion slices in a single layer on the prepared baking sheet.

6. Bake for 12 to 15 minutes or until the onions are tender and the coating is crisp. Serve.

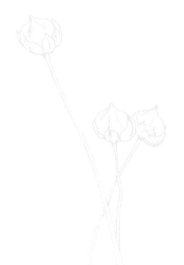

POLENTA WITH TOMATO SAUCE

1 cup (250 mL) cornmeal

4 cups (1 L) water, divided

1 tsp (5 mL) salt

⅓ cup (75 mL) ground flaxseed

¼ cup (50 mL) chopped fresh
parsley, packed

¼ cup (50 mL) grated light
Parmesan cheese

1 tsp (5 mL) whole flaxseed

2 Tbsp (25 mL) olive oil

4 cups (1 L) diced ripe tomatoes
(approximately 5 to 6 tomatoes)

salt

black pepper

olive oil for sautéing

YIELD: 8 servings

NUTRIENT VALUES PER
SERVING (2 SLICES
POLENTA WITH ¼ CUP/
50 ML SAUCE)

Calories	152
Protein	4.7 g
Carbohydrates	20.7 g
Fibre	4.0 g
Fat	6.8 g
Saturated	1.8 g
Monounsaturated	3.4 g
Polyunsaturated	1.3 g
Cholesterol	1 mg
Folate	26 mcg
Potassium	293 mg
Sodium	413 mg

1. Lightly spray an 8½- × 4½-inch (1.5 L) loaf pan with non-stick cooking spray.
2. In a bowl, combine the cornmeal with 1 cup (250 mL) of the water.
3. In a large saucepan, bring the remaining 3 cups (750 mL) of water to a boil.
4. Add the soaked cornmeal and salt to the water, stirring constantly until thickened.
5. Cover, reduce the heat to low and cook for another 10 minutes, stirring occasionally.
6. Remove from the heat and stir in the ground flaxseed, parsley and Parmesan cheese.
7. Spoon the mixture into the prepared loaf pan.
8. Sprinkle the whole flaxseed overtop. Let cool for 2 hours in the refrigerator.
9. In a medium pan over medium heat, heat the oil and diced tomatoes. Cook, stirring occasionally, until the tomatoes are soft and the sauce has thickened, about 8 minutes. Add salt and pepper to taste.
10. When the polenta is cold, cut it into sixteen ½-inch (1 cm) slices.
11. Heat a non-stick pan over medium to medium-low heat. Lightly oil it with olive oil.
12. Add a few polenta slices and fry them until they're golden, about 5 minutes on each side.
13. Keep them warm while you fry the remainder of the polenta.
14. Serve 2 slices per person with ¼ cup (50 mL) of warm tomato sauce overtop.

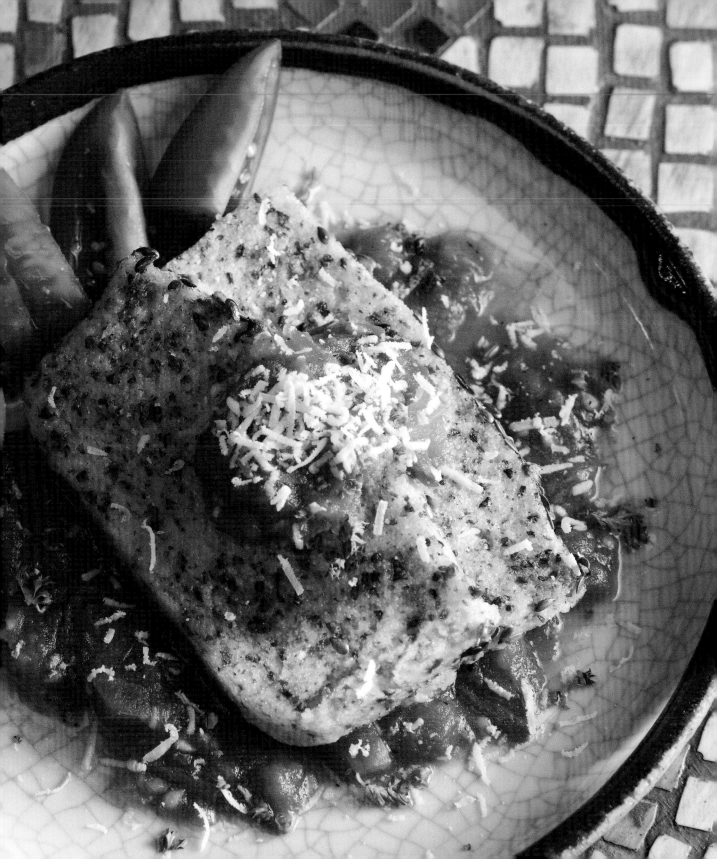

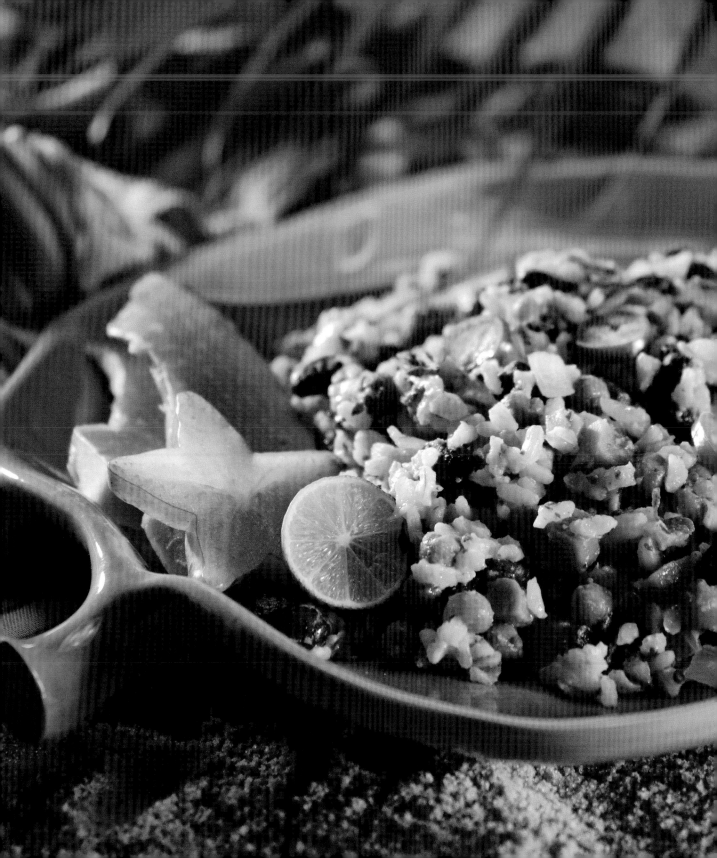

WARM CARIBBEAN BEANS & RICE

1 tsp (5 mL) canola oil

½ cup (125 mL) chopped onion

2 cloves garlic, minced

1 jalapeño pepper, minced

1½ tsp (7 mL) curry powder or paste

½ tsp (2 mL) dried thyme

½ tsp (2 mL) salt

1 cup (250 mL) cooked brown rice

1 cup (250 mL) frozen mixed peas and carrots, cooked

1 cup (250 mL) canned black beans, rinsed and drained

¼ cup (50 mL) ground flaxseed

1 Tbsp (15 mL) flaxseed oil

1 Tbsp (15 mL) fresh lime juice

YIELD: 6 servings

NUTRIENT VALUES PER SERVING (½ CUP/125 ML)

Calories	132
Protein	4.7 g
Carbohydrates	19.9 g
Fibre	5.4 g
Fat	5.7 g
Saturated	1.3 g
Monounsaturated	1.6 g
Polyunsaturated	2.6 g
Cholesterol	0 mg
Folate	12 mcg
Potassium	266 mg
Sodium	390 mg

1. In a large non-stick skillet, heat the oil over medium to medium-low heat.
2. Add the onion, garlic and jalapeño. Sauté until the onion and garlic are soft and just starting to brown, about 5 minutes.
3. Add the curry powder, thyme and salt. Stir and cook for another minute.
4. Add the cooked rice, peas and carrots, and beans. Stir.
5. Cover and heat until warmed through.
6. Stir in the ground flaxseed, flaxseed oil and lime juice. Serve immediately.

FRIED RICE

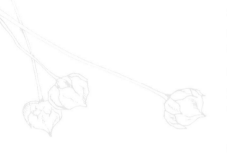

1 cup (250 mL) long-grain rice

2 cups (500 mL) water

½ tsp (2 mL) salt

2 Tbsp (25 mL) canola oil

3 eggs, well beaten

½ cup (125 mL) diced cooked ham
   or any other cooked meat

¾ cup (175 mL) frozen mixed
   vegetables (carrots, peas, corn),
   thawed under cold running water
   and drained

2 green onions, sliced ¼ inch
   (6 mm) thick

2 Tbsp (25 mL) soy sauce

½ tsp (2 mL) sesame oil

¼ cup (50 mL) whole toasted flaxseed

YIELD: 6 cups (1.5 L)

NUTRIENT VALUES PER
SERVING (1 CUP/250 ML)

Calories	266
Protein	10.9 g
Carbohydrates	32.7 g
Fibre	2.7 g
Fat	10.3 g
Saturated	1.8 g
Monounsaturated	3.7 g
Polyunsaturated	4.0 g
Cholesterol	113 mg
Folate	N/A
Potassium	259 mg
Sodium	660 mg

1. Rinse the rice well in a sieve under cold running water.
2. In a medium saucepan, bring the water and salt to a boil, add the rice and return to a boil, stirring with a fork.
3. Reduce the heat, cover and simmer slowly for 20 minutes.
4. Remove the lid and allow the steam to escape. Fluff the rice with a fork.
5. Cool, cover and refrigerate overnight.
6. In a large non-stick skillet over medium heat, heat the canola oil.
7. Add the eggs and fry them until half-cooked.
8. Add the rice, breaking up any lumps and stirring quickly to coat the rice.
9. Reduce the heat to medium-low, then add the ham, mixed vegetables and green onions.
10. Cook, turning the rice mixture gently but frequently, for 4 minutes.
11. Add the soy sauce, sesame oil and flaxseed. Reduce the heat to low, cover and cook for 3 minutes. Serve.

RICE MEDLEY

1 large red bell pepper

2 Tbsp (25 mL) ghee (see page 52)
   or olive oil

⅓ cup (75 mL) sliced green onion

1 garlic clove, diced

⅓ cup (75 mL) chopped fresh parsley

¼ cup (50 mL) chopped pitted
   black olives

3 Tbsp (45 mL) diced softened
   sun-dried tomatoes

2 Tbsp (25 mL) fresh lemon juice

¼ tsp (1 mL) salt

¼ tsp (1 mL) black pepper

4 cups (1 L) cooked white rice (hot)

¼ cup (50 mL) whole toasted golden
   flaxseed

¼ cup (50 mL) crumbled feta cheese

YIELD: 5 cups (1.25 L)

NUTRIENT VALUES PER
SERVING (1 CUP/250 ML)

Calories	348
Protein	7.3 g
Carbohydrates	54.1 g
Fibre	3.1 g
Fat	11.1 g
Saturated	2.2 g
Monounsaturated	5.0 g
Polyunsaturated	2.4 g
Cholesterol	7 mg
Folate	132 mcg
Potassium	225 mg
Sodium	357 mg

1. Preheat the broiler on high. Place the bell pepper on the broiling pan 6 inches (15 cm) from the top element. Turn frequently, every 2 minutes, until the skin is slightly charred on all sides. Remove the pepper from the pan and place it in a heat-resistant plastic bag. Seal the bag and let the pepper stand until cool to the touch. Remove the pepper from the bag and peel off the skin. Halve, core, seed and chop the pepper.

2. In a small skillet, heat the ghee. Add the green onion and sauté until soft.

3. Add the garlic and cook for 1 minute.

4. Add the parsley, olives, tomatoes, lemon juice, salt and pepper. Cook and stir for 2 minutes, until heated through.

5. Remove from the heat.

6. Add the mixture to the hot rice and toss.

7. Add the roasted pepper and flaxseed. Toss.

8. Top with the crumbled feta cheese and serve.

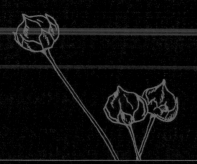
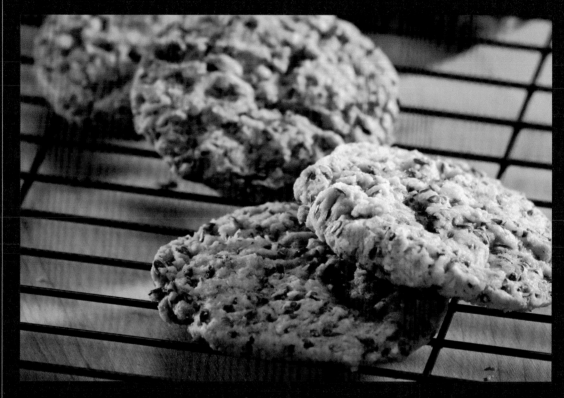
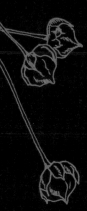

Pictured: *Farmland Cookies* (page 187)

Cookies, Cakes & Treats

Freshly baked cookies, warm from the oven, are back and better with the addition of whole and ground flaxseed or flax oil. The delightful nutty flavour and texture of flax, particularly in the Farmland Cookies or Apple Flaxseed Squares, makes it doubly easy to consume the fibre so important for the continual health of your digestive tract. We may not eat cookies as often as we used to, but when you get a hankering, these adaptations of some traditional recipes are sure to please.

Cakes, squares and bars always seem to be required for any celebration, whether it's large, small, planned or spontaneous. Flaxseed-based products store well, with many of the cakes keeping well for up to 3 months in the freezer. Flax is an excellent addition to your baking pantry staples.

We've indulged a wee bit too and included Flax Caramel, Fudge with Flax, and Chocolate Caramel Popcorn to satisfy those occasional cravings for something decadent.

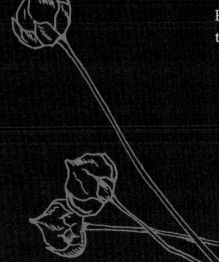

FLAX COOKIES

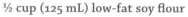

½ cup (125 mL) low-fat soy flour

¼ cup (50 mL) rice flour

¼ cup (50 mL) toasted ground
golden flaxseed

2 Tbsp (25 mL) toasted whole
golden flaxseed

¼ tsp (1 mL) salt

⅓ cup (75 mL) margarine, softened

¼ cup (50 mL) granulated sugar

¼ cup (50 mL) lightly packed
brown sugar

1 tsp (5 mL) vanilla extract

1 egg

⅓ cup (75 mL) semi-sweet chocolate
and butterscotch chips, mixed

¼ cup (50 mL) chopped pecans or
walnuts

YIELD: 20 cookies

NUTRIENT VALUES PER
SERVING (1 COOKIE)

Calories	97
Protein	2.4 g
Carbohydrates	10.0 g
Fibre	0.9 g
Fat	5.9 g
Saturated	1.4 g
Monounsaturated	2.0 g
Polyunsaturated	2.2 g
Cholesterol	9 mg
Folate	12 mcg
Potassium	102 mg
Sodium	73 mg

*Based on recipe using equal
amounts of semi-sweet and
butterscotch chips*

1. Preheat the oven to 350°F (180°C). Spray a baking sheet with non-stick
   cooking spray.
2. In a bowl, combine both flours, the ground and whole flaxseed and the salt.
3. In another bowl, beat the margarine and both sugars together.
4. Add the vanilla and egg to the margarine and sugar mixture. Beat again.
5. Add the flax mixture to the margarine and sugar mixture and stir until blended.
6. Add the chocolate and butterscotch chips and nuts and stir until combined.
7. Place the cookie dough by tablespoonfuls (approx 15 mL) 2 inches (5 cm) apart
   on the prepared baking sheet.
8. Bake for 12 minutes.
9. Remove from the oven and cool on the baking sheet for 5 minutes before
   removing to a rack to cool completely.

*These can be stored in a covered container for up to 5 days or frozen for up
to 3 months.*

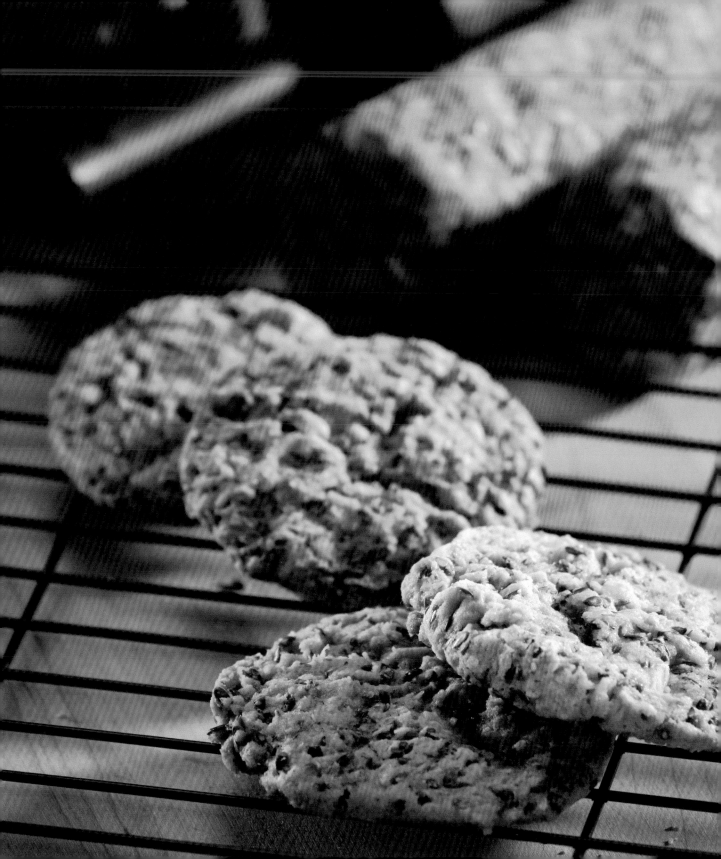

FARMLAND COOKIES

1⅓ cups (325 mL) butter

1½ cups (375 mL) lightly packed
   brown sugar

1¼ cups (300 mL) granulated sugar

2⅓ cups (575 mL) whole flaxseed

3 large eggs

1½ tsp (7 mL) vanilla extract

3⅓ cups (825 mL) unbleached
   all-purpose flour

1 Tbsp (15 mL) baking soda

3 cups (750 mL) quick-cooking oats

YIELD: 9 dozen cookies

NUTRIENT VALUES PER
SERVING (2 COOKIES)

Calories	185
Protein	3.7 g
Carbohydrates	23.9 g
Fibre	2.2 g
Fat	8.8 g
Saturated	3.5 g
Monounsaturated	2.3 g
Polyunsaturated	2.5 g
Cholesterol	25 mg
Folate	N/A
Potassium	174 mg
Sodium	134 mg

1. In a bowl, cream together the butter and both sugars, then add the flaxseed.
2. In another bowl, beat the eggs and vanilla together. Combine with the flax mixture.
3. Sift together the flour and baking soda. Mix in the oats and combine with the flax and egg mixture.
4. Form the dough into a 1½-inch (4 cm) round log. Place in the freezer and chill for 2 hours.
5. Preheat the oven to 350°F (180°C). Spray a baking sheet with non-stick cooking spray.
6. Slice the log into ¼-inch (6 mm) medallions.
7. Place on the prepared baking sheet, leaving about 2 inches (5 cm) between the cookies.
8. Bake for 13 to 15 minutes.
9. Remove from the oven and transfer to a rack to cool completely.

These can be stored in an airtight container for up to 5 days or frozen for up to 3 months.

FAVOURITE COOKIES

Flax Fact: Laying hens who are fed flax produce omega-3 eggs. These eggs contain the essential omega-3 fatty acid, alpha-linolenic acid (ALA), plus two other omega-3 fatty acids: eicosapentaenoic acid (EPA) and docosahexaenoic acid (DHA). Omega-3-enriched eggs provide about 12 times more omega-3 fatty acids than regular eggs.

¼ cup (50 mL) butter or margarine, softened

½ cup (125 mL) lightly packed brown sugar

2 Tbsp (25 mL) hot water (150°F/70°C)

1 egg

1 tsp (5 mL) vanilla extract

½ cup (125 mL) ground flaxseed

½ cup (125 mL) unbleached all-purpose flour

½ tsp (2 mL) baking soda

¼ tsp (1 mL) salt

1 cup (250 mL) old-fashioned rolled oats

½ cup (125 mL) chopped pecans

½ cup (125 mL) raisins

⅓ cup (75 mL) shredded unsweetened coconut

2 Tbsp (25 mL) whole flaxseed

YIELD: 30 cookies

NUTRIENT VALUES PER SERVING (2 COOKIES)

Calories	179
Protein	3.6 g
Carbohydrates	22.1 g
Fibre	3.4 g
Fat	9.8 g
Saturated	2.2 g
Monounsaturated	3.6 g
Polyunsaturated	3.0 g
Cholesterol	12 mg
Folate	13 mcg
Potassium	174 mg
Sodium	138 mg

SUBSTITUTE THE PECANS with your own choice of nuts or ⅓ cup (75 mL) raw sunflower seeds.

1. Preheat the oven to 375°F (190°C). Spray 2 baking sheets with non-stick cooking spray.
2. In a bowl, cream the butter and sugar.
3. Add the hot water and mix well.
4. Add the egg and vanilla and beat until light in colour.
5. Stir in the ground flaxseed, flour, baking soda and salt. Blend well.
6. Stir in the oats, pecans, raisins, coconut and whole flaxseed.
7. Drop by level tablespoonfuls (approx 15 mL) 2 inches (5 cm) apart on the prepared baking sheets.
8. Lightly press down the cookies with the bottom of a floured glass.
9. Bake for 8 to 10 minutes or until golden brown.
10. Remove from the oven. Remove the cookies from the baking sheets and allow to cool completely on a rack.

These can be stored in an airtight container for up to 3 days or frozen for up to 3 months.

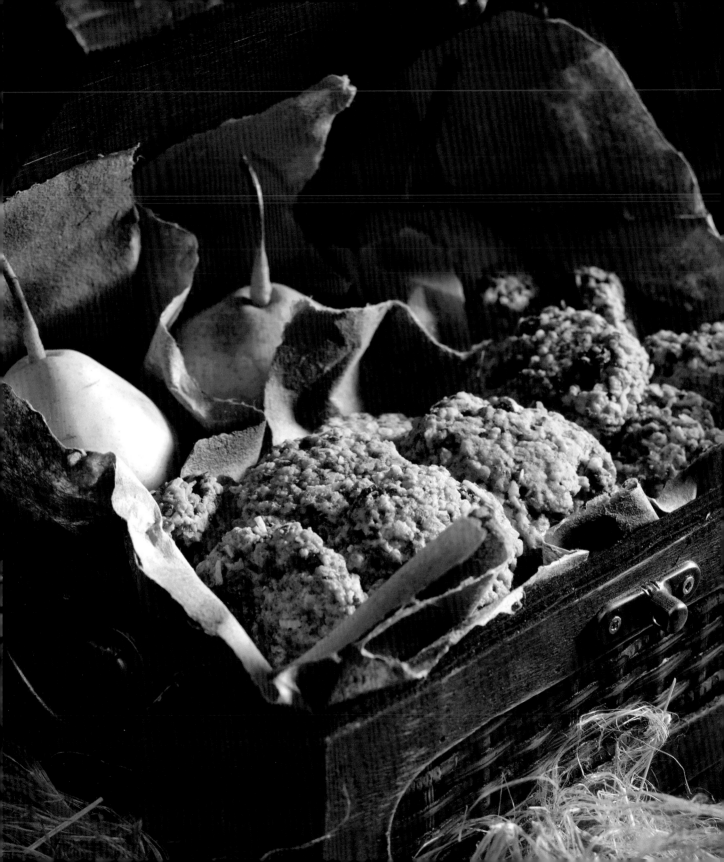

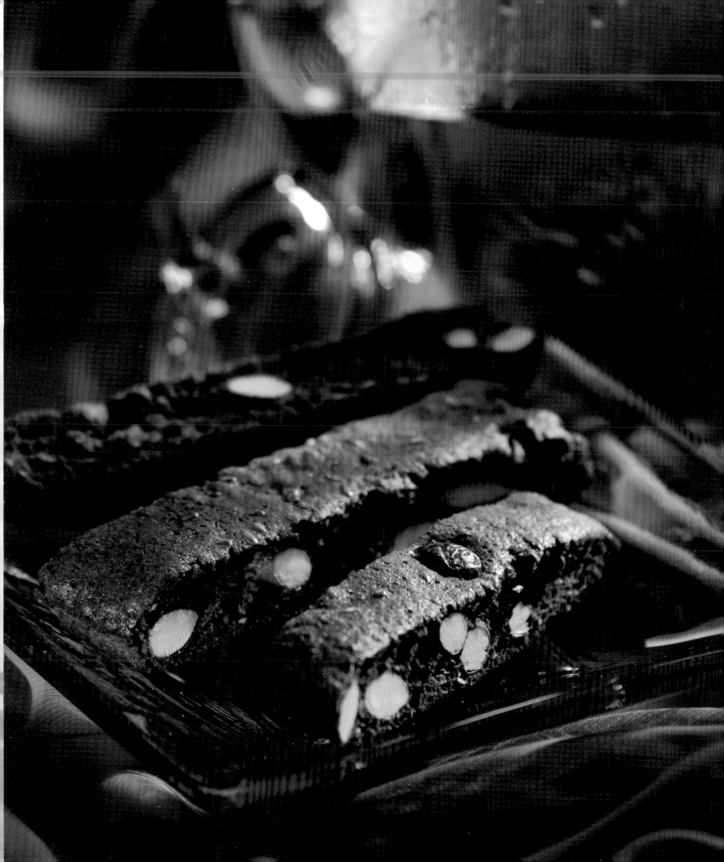

BISCOTTI

½ cup (125 mL) liquid honey

½ cup (125 mL) water

4 egg whites

2 cups (500 mL) unbleached
   all-purpose flour

⅔ cup (150 mL) granulated sugar

1½ tsp (7 mL) baking powder

1½ tsp (7 mL) baking soda

¼ tsp (1 mL) salt

2 Tbsp (25 mL) ground cinnamon

1½ cups (375 mL) whole unblanched
   almonds

½ cup (125 mL) whole flaxseed

⅔ cup (150 mL) cran-raisins
   (optional)

YIELD: 50 slices

NUTRIENT VALUES PER
SERVING (2 SLICES)

Calories	145
Protein	3.6 g
Carbohydrates	22.0 g
Fibre	2.5 g
Fat	5.5 g
Saturated	0.5 g
Monounsaturated	3.0 g
Polyunsaturated	1.6 g
Cholesterol	0 mg
Folate	29 mcg
Potassium	112 mg
Sodium	126 mg

FOR A CHOCOLATE
BISCOTTI, use 2 Tbsp
(25 mL) unsweetened cocoa
powder instead of the cinnamon and mini chocolate
chips instead of the cran-
raisins.

1. Preheat the oven to 350°F (180°C). Line a baking sheet with parchment paper.
2. In a bowl, whisk together the honey, water and egg whites.
3. In another bowl, sift together the flour, sugar, baking powder, baking soda, salt and cinnamon. Stir in the almonds, flaxseed and cran-raisins (if using).
4. Mix the dry ingredients into the liquid ingredients until just blended.
5. Spread the dough on the prepared baking sheet to make 2 loaves, each 4 inches (10 cm) wide. Smooth the edges slightly.
6. Bake for 40 to 45 minutes or until dark and firm. Remove from the oven.
7. Reduce the oven temperature to 250°F (120°C).
8. Cut the loaves into ½-inch (1 cm) slices. Place the slices on the prepared baking sheet and bake for another 10 to 15 minutes, or until very crisp.
9. Turn off the oven and cool the biscotti in the oven for several hours with the oven door slightly open.

These can be stored in an airtight container in the refrigerator for up to 1 week.

RASPBERRY SCOTCH SQUARES

1 cup (250 mL) unbleached
  all-purpose flour
¾ cup (175 mL) lightly packed
  brown sugar
½ cup (125 mL) ground flaxseed
1 tsp (5 mL) baking powder
¼ tsp (1 mL) salt

½ cup (125 mL) butter or margarine
1½ cups (375 mL) old-fashioned
  rolled oats
2 Tbsp (25 mL) whole flaxseed
1 cup (250 mL) raspberry jam
⅓ cup (75 mL) sliced almonds

YIELD: one 9- × 13-inch
(23 × 33 cm) baking pan
(18 squares)

NUTRIENT VALUES PER
SERVING (2 SQUARES)

Calories	242
Protein	4.6 g
Carbohydrates	37.3 g
Fibre	3.5 g
Fat	9.2 g
Saturated	1.6 g
Monounsaturated	3.7 g
Polyunsaturated	3.4 g
Cholesterol	0 mg
Folate	30 mcg
Potassium	165 mg
Sodium	127 mg

1. Preheat the oven to 375°F (190°C). Lightly spray a 9- × 13-inch (23 × 33 cm) baking pan with non-stick cooking spray.
2. In a medium bowl, combine the flour, sugar, ground flaxseed, baking powder and salt. Stir well.
3. Add the butter. Cut it with a knife into smaller pieces, then use your fingers to rub it into the dry mixture until crumbly.
4. Stir in the oats and whole flaxseed.
5. Press two-thirds of the crumb mixture into the prepared pan.
6. Spread with jam.
7. Add the almonds to the remaining crumbs and sprinkle over the jam. Pat lightly.
8. Bake for 30 to 35 minutes or until golden.
9. Remove to a cooling rack to cool in the pan.
10. When cool, cut into 3 rows lengthwise and 6 rows crosswise.

These can be stored in an airtight container for up to 3 days or frozen for up to 3 months.

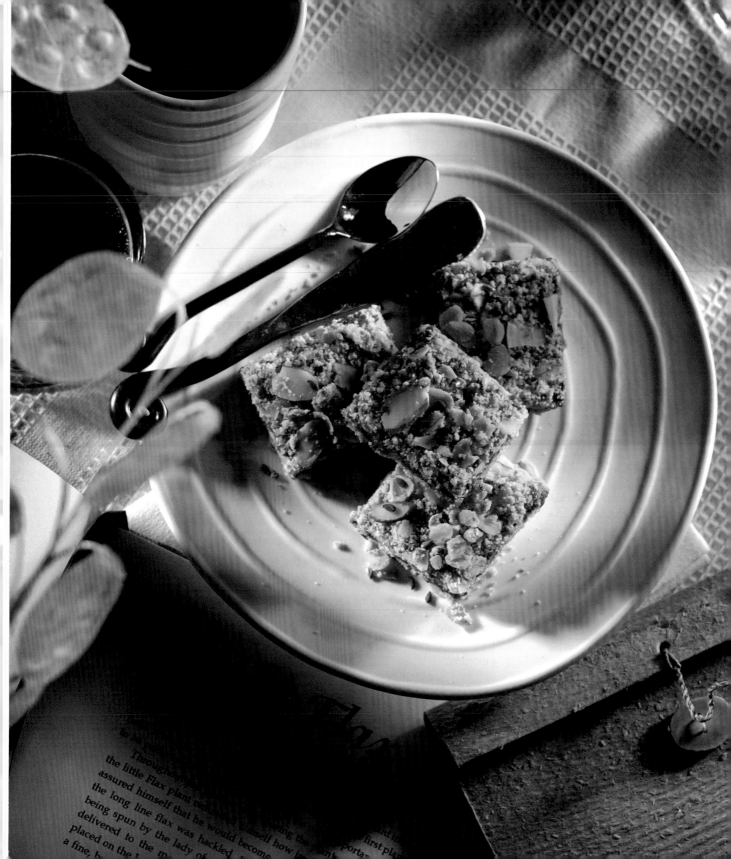

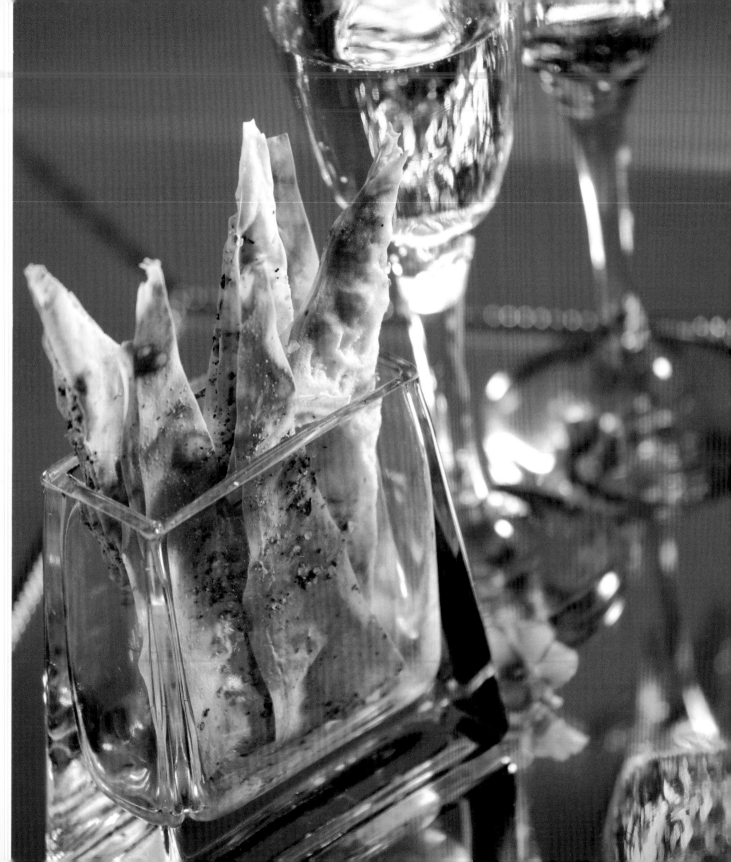

TURBINADO SUGAR &
BLACK PEPPER PHYLLO SHARDS

¼ cup (50 mL) ground flaxseed

¼ cup (50 mL) turbinado (raw) sugar

1 Tbsp (15 mL) whole flaxseed

1 Tbsp (15 mL) cracked or coarsely
    ground black pepper

4 sheets phyllo pastry (12 × 16 inches/
    30 × 40 cm each)

3 Tbsp (45 mL) melted butter,
    for brushing

YIELD: 32 triangles

NUTRIENT VALUES PER
SERVING (2 TRIANGLES)

Calories	212
Protein	2.8 g
Carbohydrates	17.6 g
Fibre	1.2 g
Fat	15.0 g
Saturated	3.5 g
Monounsaturated	3.6 g
Polyunsaturated	7.2 g
Cholesterol	6 mg
Folate	15 mcg
Potassium	51 mg
Sodium	102 mg

TURBINADO SUGAR is
sometimes also known as
raw sugar. It has a delicate
molasses or brown-sugar
taste, and its blond-coloured
crystals are dry, coarse and
noticeably larger than granulated sugar crystals.

1. Preheat the oven to 400°F (200°C). Line a baking sheet with parchment paper.

2. In a small bowl, combine the ground flaxseed, sugar, whole flaxseed and pepper.

3. On the prepared baking sheet, place 1 sheet of phyllo. Brush the top with 2 tsp (10 mL) of the melted butter and sprinkle generously with the flaxseed mixture. Repeat this process twice.

4. Top with the fourth sheet of phyllo and brush it with the remaining butter.

5. Use a sharp knife to cut the sheets in half crosswise. Then cut at 2-inch (5 cm) intervals to form sixteen 2- × 6-inch (5 × 15 cm) rectangles. Cut each rectangle diagonally to form 32 triangles.

6. Bake for 12 minutes, until the triangles are golden, crisp and dry to the touch.

7. Remove from the oven and let cool in the pan for 5 minutes before removing to a rack to cool completely.

These can be stored in an airtight container for up to 5 days.

FRUIT & BERRY COBBLER

Flax Fact: According to the American Dietetic Association, dietary fibre can have a "significant impact" on the prevention of obesity, cardiovascular disease and Type 2 diabetes.

Flaxseed is stunningly high in dietary fibre, with 28% fibre and a perfect ratio of soluble (20 to 40%) to insoluble (60% to 80%) fibre.

Filling

5 cups (1.25 L) sliced fruit (apple, peach, pear)

2 Tbsp (25 mL) fresh lemon juice

juice of 1 orange

2 cups (500 mL) fresh or frozen raspberries, strawberries, blueberries or Saskatoon berries

⅓ cup (75 mL) granulated sugar

3 Tbsp (45 mL) cornstarch

2 Tbsp (25 mL) ground flaxseed

½ tsp (2 mL) ground cinnamon

Biscuits

1 cup (250 mL) unbleached all-purpose flour

⅓ cup (75 mL) ground flaxseed

¼ cup (50 mL) granulated sugar

grated zest of 1 orange

1½ tsp (7 mL) baking powder

1 tsp (5 mL) baking soda

¼ tsp (1 mL) salt

2 Tbsp (25 mL) butter or margarine

½ cup (125 mL) buttermilk (see page 18)

Topping

¼ cup (50 mL) chopped walnuts or pecans, or sliced almonds

2 Tbsp (25 mL) brown sugar

1 Tbsp (15 mL) whole flaxseed

¼ tsp (1 mL) ground cinnamon

IF USING PEACHES, peel them before using them in the recipe.

1. Preheat the oven to 375°F (190°C). Lightly spray a 12-cup (3 L) casserole dish with non-stick cooking spray.
2. For the filling, in a large bowl, toss the fruit slices with the lemon and orange juice.
3. Add the berries, sugar, cornstarch, ground flaxseed and cinnamon. Stir.
4. Turn into the prepared casserole dish. Bake for 15 minutes, then stir.
5. For the biscuits, in a medium bowl, combine the flour, ground flaxseed, sugar, orange zest, baking powder, baking soda and salt. Cut in the butter. Rub the mixture lightly with your fingertips until it resembles coarse crumbs.

Continued on page 220 . . .

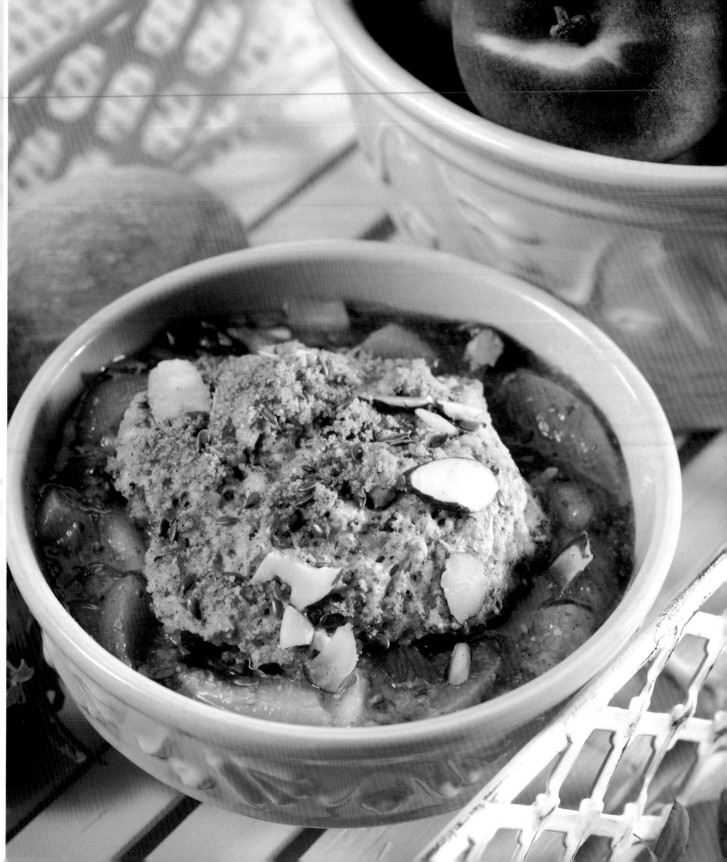

CHOCOLATE CARAMEL POPCORN

20 cups (5 L) popped popcorn

1 cup (250 mL) lightly packed
  brown sugar

¾ cup (175 mL) granulated sugar

¾ cup (175 mL) butter

½ cup (125 mL) corn syrup

1 tsp (5 mL) vanilla extract

½ tsp (2 mL) baking soda

2 cups (500 mL) milk chocolate chips

½ cup (125 mL) whole toasted
  golden flaxseed

½ cup (125 mL) toasted slivered
  almonds

YIELD: 20 cups (5 L)

NUTRIENT VALUES PER
SERVING (¾ CUP/175 ML)

Calories	406
Protein	4.7 g
Carbohydrates	56.4 g
Fibre	4.2 g
Fat	20.0 g
Saturated	10.2 g
Monounsaturated	6.5 g
Polyunsaturated	2.4 g
Cholesterol	34 mg
Folate	18 mcg
Potassium	234 mg
Sodium	174 mg

1. Preheat the oven to 250°F (120°C). Spray two 9- × 13-inch (23 × 33 cm) baking pans with non-stick cooking spray.
2. Divide the popcorn between the prepared pans.
3. In a medium saucepan, combine both the sugars, the butter and the corn syrup.
4. Cook over medium to medium-high heat until the mixture comes to a full boil, stirring occasionally.
5. Reduce the temperature to medium-low. Continue cooking without stirring until a candy thermometer displays 234°F (112°C).
6. Remove from the heat. Stir in the vanilla and baking soda. Be careful when you do this as the mixture will bubble vigorously.
7. Pour the caramel mixture over the popcorn.
8. Sprinkle the chocolate chips, flaxseed and almonds over the popcorn. Stir to coat the popcorn.
9. Bake for 45 minutes, stirring the popcorn mixture every 15 minutes.
10. Remove from the oven and transfer the popcorn to wax paper.
11. Cool completely.

This can be stored in an airtight container for up to 5 days.

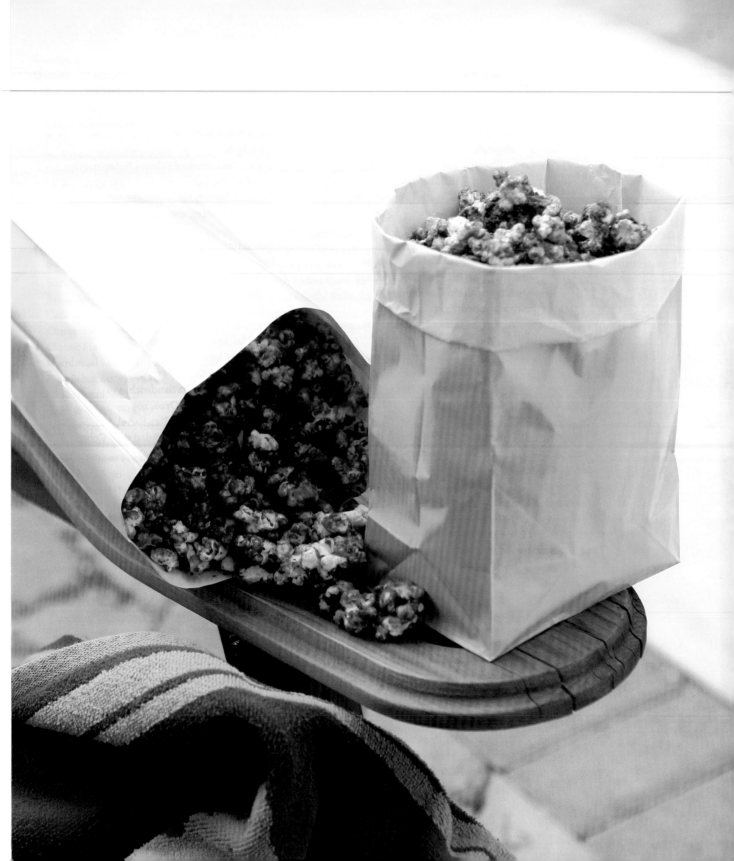

SOURCES FOR FLAX FACTS

Websites

Agricultural Marketing Resource Center,
The. www.agmrc.org/commodities__
products/grains__oilseeds/flax.cfm.

Ameriflax. www.ameriflax.com.

FatsforHealth.com. EFA library.
www.fatsforhealth.com/library/.

Flax Council of Canada.
www.flaxcouncil.ca.

Saskatchewan Flax Development
Commission. www.saskflax.com.

Books and periodicals

McGee, Harold. 1984. *On Food and
Cooking: The science and lore of the
kitchen.* (Rev. ed.) New York:
Scribner.

Riotte, Louise. 1998. *Carrots Love
Tomatoes: Secrets of companion
planting for successful gardening.*
North Adams, MA: Storey Publishing.

Saskatchewan Flax Development Commis-
sion and Aamir Asgarali. February 2007.
Flaxseed: Situation and Outlook.
Bi-weekly Bulletin 20, no. 3.